ESSENTIAL OILS
NATURAL REMEDIES

WHAT AILS YOU?

CONGESTION

There's no need to resort to syrups and pills when you have eucalyptus essential oil. Rub a few drops of it on your hands and cup them over your face before inhaling, or inhale the scent directly from the bottle, for rapid congestion relief. SEE PAGE 108

HEADACHE

Hold off on the ibuprofen, and massage a drop of peppermint essential oil into your temples to ease the throbbing. SEE PAGE 143

INSOMNIA

Instead of taking sleeping pills, sprinkle lavender essential oil on your pillowcase to help you nod off. SEE PAGE 159

Essential oils offer simple, effective, natural remedies that treat the root cause of disease, and not symptoms. Say goodbye to over-prescribed modern drug-based therapies, and experience for yourself the timeless healing power of essential oils. An A-Z list of essential oils healing recipes begins on PAGE 64

Essential Oils

THE COMPLETE A-Z REFERENCE *of* ESSENTIAL OILS *for* HEALTH *and* HEALING

Natural Remedies

ALTHEA
PRESS

CONTENTS

CHAPTER FIVE

Nature's Pharmacy of Essential Oils 270

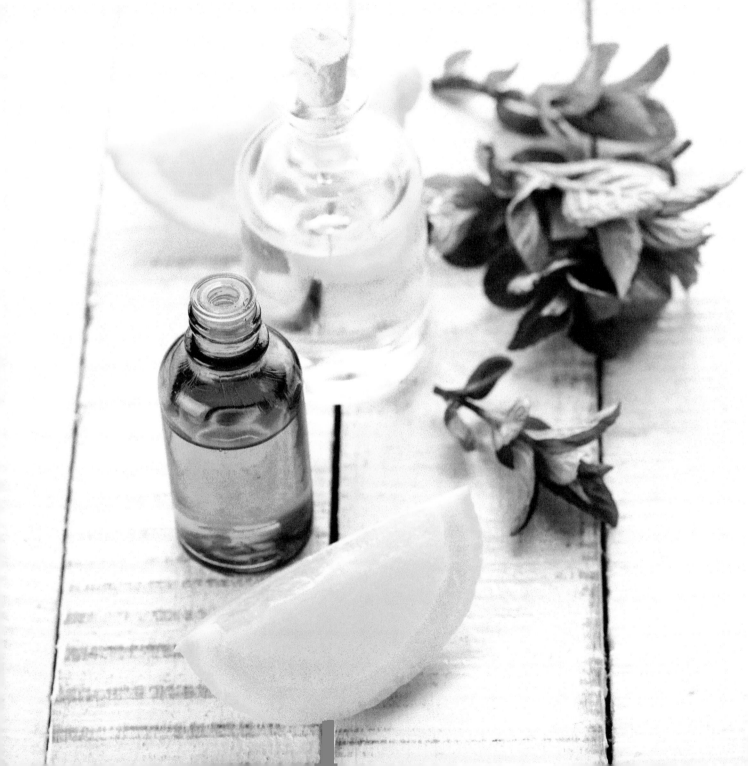

INTRODUCTION

Modern medicine saves countless lives each day. With it come such marvels as medical imaging, an unprecedented understanding of human genetics, incredible trauma treatments and surgical techniques, and much more. Even so, conventional medicine remains ineffective in many areas of our health and healing; invasive treatments commonly cause severe side effects, and preventive care is too often overlooked. Where many mainstream treatments fail, natural medicine often excels. Essential oils play a vital role in natural or complementary medicine, and because they are safe, simple to administer, and noninvasive, they are ideal for inclusion in nearly any self-care plan.

Fortunately, mainstream medicine and modern techniques aren't the only options available to us. For thousands of years, essential oils and other natural remedies were the only medicines available, proving themselves time and again in daily life. What worked for healers past can and should work just as well for us today.

Every aspiring essential oil practitioner can benefit from a handbook, but herbal compendiums can be confusing, and many books on essential oils are equally mind-boggling. This one aims to inform you while being easier to navigate and simpler to use than any other guide. With practical, factual, in-depth information on using essential oils to treat over 170 common maladies, this on-demand reference has been designed so you can find the information you want when you need it.

If you're new to using essential oils, begin by reading Chapter One, which contains a comprehensive introduction to essential oils and aromatherapy.

- What are essential oils, and how are they produced?
- What is the difference between fragrance oils and essential oils?
- What are the safest ways to use essential oils?

In addition to answering these and many other questions, you'll also learn about the basic tools required to get started with essential oils.

Look in Chapter Four to find the remedies that will bring relief. This section contains remedies for a wide range of common health complaints, arranged in alphabetical order for easy navigation. Here you will find details about why each remedy works along with applicable safety precautions and other vital information. For a quick page reference, turn to the Ailments Index on page 437 of this book.

Chapter Five provides an alphabetized list of 75 of the most useful essential oils. Included are critical facts about each essential oil, including its common name, Latin name, complete information concerning its medicinal use, and detailed information for blending it with other essential oils to enhance its efficacy. You'll find label safety warnings, as well, so you'll know which essential oils are safe for you to use and which you should avoid.

In the chapters ahead, you will:

- Gain the understanding you need to start using essential oils right away.
- Learn the facts about essential oils use and treatment. Medical, scientific, and safety facts are found throughout the book, and are formatted for ease of identification.
- Receive easy-to-follow instructions for treating common illnesses and minor injuries with a variety of basic but powerful and effective homemade remedies.

People turn to essential oils for one, two, or perhaps several reasons—to take charge of their own health, to explore natural alternatives to pharmaceuticals, to save money, and to ensure preparedness in the face of emergencies and disasters. Whether your goal is to gain expertise in using essential oils or to simply improve your ability to care for your own health, this book will be an indispensable resource.

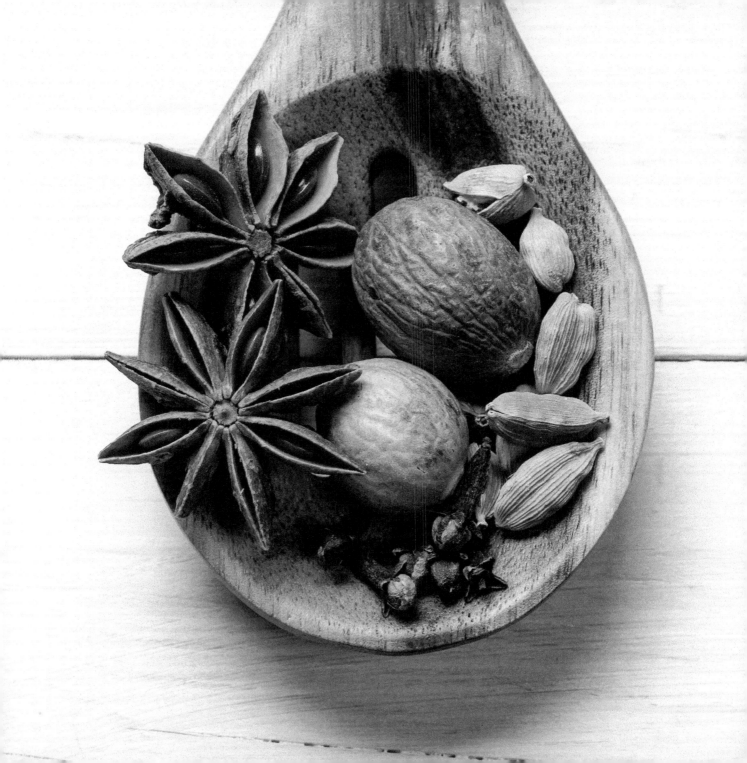

1

LET PLANTS BE THY MEDICINE

Essential oils are beneficial to
the body, the mind and spirit,
and even your wallet.

Before factories produced medicines, people relied on natural remedies made with plants. Essential oils are among the most powerful healing agents the natural environment has to offer. Derived from the leaves, roots, flowers, and bark of plants, essential oils are aromatic compounds that form deep within plant cells, providing plants with protection from disease, deterring hungry insects, and making plants more appealing to pollinators. Essential oils likewise offer the most natural way for you to prevent and treat ailments of your own, as well as enhance health and promote total well-being. These oils were sacred to ancient Egyptians and central to India's Ayurveda practices, and they were used extensively by Roman and Greek physicians, who ultimately shared their knowledge with scholars from other parts of the globe.

A BRIEF HISTORY

The pharmaceutical industry as we know it today got its start in the Middle Ages. The first documented drugstore was opened in Baghdad in the year 754, and such stores gained popularity throughout the Islamic world in subsequent years. Formularies and herb shops selling remedies of all kinds were common throughout Medieval Europe and Asia. The late 1800s saw pharmaceutical companies—including Parke-Davis, Squibb, Lilly, The Upjohn Company, Searle, and Abbott—spring up in the United States. Other pioneering drug companies included Pfizer, Bayer, and Johnson & Johnson. Many medicines produced by these companies were, and still are, plant-based; many others are synthetic.

By the dawn of the 20th century, many people stopped using whole-plant remedies and essential oils in favor of convenient preparations offered by drug manufacturers. Important life-saving discoveries, including penicillin and insulin, changed the face of health care by the end of the 1930s, and plants as medicine were largely relegated to the realm of folk medicine.

Drugs were in short supply during the Second World War, when Dr. Jean Valnet made a discovery that reminded people of the power of essential oils. After running out of antibiotics, he began to use eucalyptus essential oil as a bactericide, saving lives as a result of his willingness to step outside the pharmaceutical box.

Prescription drugs and over-the-counter (OTC) medications are often pricey. A 2010 AARP study showed a 41 percent increase in the cost of name-brand drugs during the five-year period between 2004 and 2009. Retail prices have continued to escalate since then, with the cost of 73 popular brands increasing by a shocking 73 percent between 2007 and 2014.

You, too, can take advantage of nature's pharmacy of healing plants rather than relying solely upon modern medicine. Essential oils offer versatility, portability, potency, and safety—something that cannot be said of all plant-based remedies.

WHAT ARE ESSENTIAL OILS?

Pure essential oils are highly concentrated compounds that have been pressed or distilled from plants. Unlike *fixed oils* such as vegetable cooking oils, they do not have a fatty or oily component. Called essential because they carry the distinctive fragrance or essence of the plant or plant part from which they are made, these oils are used primarily for aromatherapy, and also for scenting soaps, candles, and other products. Some essential oils, including peppermint and cinnamon, are used for flavoring products such as candy and toothpaste, and others are used in formulating household cleaners.

BASIC ESSENTIAL OIL TERMINOLOGY

As you make your way through this book and other resources, you'll notice terminology that may be unfamiliar. Here are short explanations of some of the most frequently-used vocabulary. (For additional terms, see the glossary on page 423.)

- **aromatherapy:** The practice of using natural aromatic substances, including essential oils, for their physical and psychological therapeutic benefits.
- **botanical name:** A specific Latin name that distinguishes variants of plants that share the same common name.
- **carrier oil:** An oil used for diluting an essential oil prior to use.
- **common name:** A plant's everyday name.
- **dilution:** The act of diluting an essential oil with a carrier oil at a specific ratio.
- **diffuser:** A device used for releasing essential oil molecules into the air. Various models are available commercially.
- **food grade:** An essential oil considered safe for use in food by the FDA.
- **fragrance:** An aroma. Products labeled as fragrances are derived by synthetic means and are not essential oils.
- **herbal:** Pertaining to plants.
- **insoluble:** A substance that is not capable of being dissolved in liquid such as water.
- **neat:** Undiluted. Some essential oils are suitable for using neat, while others are not. As you delve deeper into the world of essential oils, you will notice that some practitioners are much more conservative than others, advising readers not to use undiluted essential oils. The choice is yours.
- **pendant:** A necklace made from a variety of materials, such as glass or terra cotta, that you can add your favorite essential oil to and wear throughout the day.
- **rectification:** The process of redistilling certain essential oils to rid them of undesirable constituents.
- **single oil:** An essential oil from only one plant species.
- **soluble:** A substance that is capable of being dissolved in liquid such as water.
- **synergistic blend:** A combination of essential oils that offers more benefits than the same essential oils applied singly.
- **synthetic:** A substance that is unnatural or created in a laboratory. Many commercially produced drugs are synthetic.
- **volatile:** A substance that is unstable and evaporates easily.

THE BENEFITS OF ESSENTIAL OILS

Essential oils are beneficial to the body, the mind and spirit, and even your wallet. They are used to treat conditions ranging from anxiety to shingles as well as to increase overall well-being in myriad ways, many of which are discussed in-depth in subsequent chapters.

- ***All essential oils are adaptogens.*** An adaptogen is a natural substance that promotes a balancing reaction in the body, improving its ability to overcome stress and fatigue that contribute to disease. Some adaptogens improve healing, some suppress infections, and some accelerate recovery from illness or hasten healing after an injury. Numerous studies have proven that adaptogens have a normalizing effect on all of the body's functions without causing disruptions or side effects.

- ***Most essential oils are cost-effective.*** Essential oils are a less costly alternative to drugs produced by pharmaceutical companies. Lavender essential oil, for example, is a popular natural sleep aid and costs less per dose than most commercial sleep aids. It is also a phenomenal substitute for petroleum-based first aid ointments. Peppermint and eucalyptus essential oils are excellent decongestants despite costing just a few pennies per dose. When you choose to use natural botanical compounds to combat common health complaints, you save money instead of contributing to drug company profits.

- ***Many essential oils are analgesics.*** An analgesic is a substance that acts directly on the nervous system to subdue pain. Clove, peppermint, birch, and thyme essential oils are a few examples of natural, effective analgesics.

Stop menstrual pain with thyme essential oil. Thyme outperformed ibuprofen in combating menstrual pain, according to a 2014 triple-blind clinical study conducted at Babol University of Medical Sciences in Iran. As proven by researchers from Nara Women's University in Japan, thyme essential oil inhibits the COX-2 enzyme, which is partly responsible for the body's pain-producing inflammatory process.

- ***Many essential oils are anti-inflammatory.*** Inflammation is an important part of the body's natural defense system, promoting healing after exposure to toxins or following an injury. Typical signs of inflammation include swelling, redness, and pain at the affected site. Bergamot, clove, eucalyptus, and thyme essential oils are renowned for their anti-inflammatory properties. In many cases, you will find it's not necessary to take OTC drugs, since these oils are capable of providing effective relief from inflammation—without the addition of toxic chemicals.

- ***Some essential oils are antiseptics.*** An antiseptic is an antimicrobial substance that, when applied to living tissue, reduces the risk of infection. Clove, lavender, and tea tree essential oils are among the most powerful of all-natural antiseptics. Not only are these wonderful for use in treating minor injuries, they are also useful for creating natural cleaning products.

- ***Some essential oils promote relaxation and relieve stress.*** For many, stress is a part of daily life. If you've ever been overly stressed, you know how negativity can take over, creating chaos and tension while leading to physical symptoms such as headaches, indigestion, and even itchy, red rashes. Peppermint, rosemary, and ylang-ylang essential oils are excellent choices for stress relief. Others are excellent for promoting relaxation, enhancing meditation, and hastening sleep.

Whether you are suffering from a throbbing headache, sore muscles, dermatitis, fatigue, or another irritating or painful condition, it is likely that an effective essential oil remedy exists. Because essential oils work by targeting the cause of a problem rather than simply addressing symptoms, you are likely to experience rapid relief and steady improvement.

HOW ESSENTIAL OILS ARE PRODUCED

Because plants are complex, essential oils are extracted using several different techniques. Like wine making, essential oil production is both an art and a science. All methods are important, and the value of the finished product depends greatly on the distiller's experience and on the oil's intended application.

Steam Distillation

Steam distillation is the most common method for producing essential oils. There are two types of steam distillation:

1. Steam is injected into a tightly sealed chamber that holds raw plant materials. As the steam strikes the plants, the heat causes small internal sacs to burst. These sacs hold the essential oil, and are the same ones that rupture when you rub an aromatic plant such as lavender, rosemary, or sage between your fingers and catch a strong whiff of its fragrance. Essential oil molecules are minuscule, and are easily transported out of the chamber and into a chilled condenser by the airborne steam. After collection is complete, the essential oil and water are separated.
2. The whole plant is suspended above a large container of boiling water. The rising steam collects the essential oils and continues upward, where a receptacle catches it and pushes it through a separator. In both methods, the remaining water is normally reserved. Called hydrosol, it is delightfully scented and is used to add fragrance to linen sprays, perfumes, and body care products such as body lotion and facial moisturizer.

Several types of essential oil are best when produced via distillation, as some components are released only after a certain amount of exposure to gentle heat. For example, German chamomile must be steam distilled to allow for the release its anti-inflammatory component, chamulzine. According to the Montana State University's Northwestern Agricultural Research Center, this compound gives the essential oil its characteristic blue color.

Carbon Dioxide Extraction

There are two primary methods by which essential oils are commonly extracted: carbon dioxide (CO_2) distillation and supercritical CO_2 distillation.

- **Carbon dioxide distillation**, or CO_2 extraction, uses carbon dioxide to carry the essential oil away from the raw plant material. In this method, carbon dioxide is chilled to between 35 and 55 degrees Fahrenheit before being blasted through the plant material. This is much like cold-pressing (see page 22) in that it yields pure essential oils that have not been even slightly altered by exposure to heat.
- In **supercritical CO_2 distillation**, the carbon dioxide is heated to 87 degrees Fahrenheit before being blown through the plant matter at a much higher speed. Under these intense conditions, the CO_2 is transformed into a heavy vapor that rapidly carries the essential oil away from the inert plant material. As the CO_2 is warm rather than hot, the resulting essential oil is pure and unaltered.

Many manufacturers do not distinguish between cold CO_2 distillation and supercritical CO_2 distillation when labeling the essential oils they produce, since both processes produce excellent finished products. Frankincense and myrrh essential oils are usually produced via CO_2 distillation, as are other spicy-smelling oils such as clove, black pepper, and ginger.

Some producers pride themselves on offering two additional types of CO_2-distilled essential oils: CO_2 totals and CO_2 selects.

- **CO_2 totals** are so named because they contain large amounts of plant matter, including resins, waxes, and color compounds, which are normally discarded during the manufacturing process. CO_2 totals cannot normally be poured without being warmed; their consistency is typically pasty or waxy.
- **CO_2 selects** are thicker than most other essential oils because a portion of the plant's natural waxes, resins, and color compounds are included in the finished product. These essential oils may normally be poured without prior warming.

Both CO_2 total and select essential oil are more highly concentrated than standard essential oil. Manufacturers typically recommend that you dilute them by 50 to 65 percent before use. If you happen to choose CO_2 total or select essential oils, ensure efficacy and safety by following the producer's specific recommendations for use.

Cold-Pressing

The process of cold-pressing, or expression, is used exclusively for obtaining essential oils from citrus fruits. This simple method involves placing the aromatic portion of the fruit's rind in a press at 120 degrees Fahrenheit to extract the essential oil that gives citrus fruits their characteristic scents.

Enfleurage

Hot enfleurage, which calls for the combination of fat or fatty oil with whole flowers, is the oldest-known method of essential oil extraction. Still used by some exclusive perfume manufacturers, the process involves placing blossoms in a shallow layer of warmed fatty oil that absorbs the essential oils from the petals. As the flowers wilt, they are replaced with new ones until the oil has been completely saturated with essential oil. The essential oil is then extracted with a solvent such as alcohol, and the remaining fat or oil is used to impart fragrance to soap and other products.

Solvent Extraction

Essential oils extracted with the help of chemical solvents such as methylene chloride, hexane, or benzene are called *absolutes*. In this method, the solvent is used in place of water or CO_2. Much of the solvent evaporates during the initial phase of extraction, and the remainder is spun off in a centrifuge or removed via a vacuum. However, solvent extraction leaves minute traces of the extraction chemicals in the essential oil, and noted aromatherapist Robert Tisserand points out that there is some concern about whether these minute traces are acceptable for use in aromatherapy.

UNDERSTANDING AROMATHERAPY

The word *aroma* is derived from the Greek word for *spice* and is broadly used to denote fragrance. Aromatherapy is a form of alternative medicine that draws upon the healing power of plants, with a strong focus on essential oils. In aromatherapy, these oils are used for improving physical and mental health as well as for positively influencing mood and cognitive function.

The term *aromatherapy* is a bit of a misnomer, giving the impression that this form of medicine is based solely upon scent. Rather, in aromatherapy, essential oils are inhaled for the physical and psychological benefits that occur as the oil's molecules stimulate the brain. They are also applied topically, allowing for absorption through the skin and into the bloodstream. Because essential oils vary in potency, it is vital that you follow instructions for dilution prior to use. In addition, more is not necessarily better; a small amount of essential oil is usually plenty.

Because aromatherapy is noninvasive, it is often suitable for use alongside other forms of therapy. Holistic practitioners, who seek to treat the whole patient rather than focusing solely on the symptoms and the illness, are pioneers in using aromatherapy in conjunction with Western medical treatments, homeopathic remedies, herbal medicine, Reiki, meditation, and more. Like these practitioners, you may do the same, using aromatherapy to complement other treatments.

Although merchandise that contains synthetic ingredients is often marketed as aromatherapy, products that contain artificial components of any kind are frowned upon by professionals.

Always read product ingredient lists. The Food and Drug Administration (FDA) does not regulate the use of the term aromatherapy on product labels or in product advertising. Any product, even one containing synthetic ingredients, can be marketed as suitable for use in aromatherapy. Check ingredients carefully when choosing products containing essential oils for holistic use.

ESSENTIALS OF ESSENTIAL OILS: 15 THINGS YOU SHOULD KNOW

As you delve deeper into the world of essential oils, you'll discover that the amount of information available can be overwhelming. Keep these basic facts and guidelines in mind as you learn.

1. **Essential oils aren't oils at all.** Despite their appearance and that *oil* is part of their name, the substances we call essential oils are not technically oils, as they do not contain fatty acids. Instead, essential oils are concentrated organic elements with potent medicinal qualities.

2. **Fragrance oils are not essential oils.** Even if a bottle is labeled as *natural fragrance*, it is not an essential oil if it also contains the terms *fragrance oil, fragrance,* or *perfume*.

3. **Essential oils are highly concentrated.** One hundred pounds of lavender produce a single pound of lavender essential oil, and two tons of Bulgarian roses produce just one pound of rose essential oil. A single drop of essential oil may contain the power of several plants.

4. **If you are pregnant, skip essential oils altogether during the first trimester.** In addition, many essential oils are emmenagogues, which stimulate blood flow in the uterus, bringing on menstruation. Specific safety details about all essential oils are included in Chapter Five.

5. **Keep essential oils out of reach of children.** While certain essential oils are ideal for use by everyone in the family, many are not suitable for use by children, and several are toxic if swallowed.

6. **Conduct a patch test prior to using an unfamiliar essential oil.** To prevent painful skin irritation, conduct a patch test prior to applying an unfamiliar essential oil or a product that contains something you haven't used in the past. Combine a single drop of the essential oil with ½ teaspoon of the carrier oil of your choice, then rub it on the inside portion of your upper arm. Wait a few hours to ensure no itching or redness develops.

7. **If you are allergic to a plant, you are allergic to its essential oil.** Since essential oil is a highly concentrated form of a plant, if you are allergic to the plant, such as chamomile, roses, or thyme, avoid using the essential oil in any capacity.

8. **Watch out for adulteration.** When purchasing an essential oil from an unfamiliar source, check to ensure it is pure before using it for aromatherapy. To do this, place a single drop of the oil on a piece of paper. It should evaporate within an hour at the most, and it should not leave a ring of oil behind. This test works for all oils except myrrh and patchouli, and absolutes such as jasmine, rose, and vanilla. Always purchase essential oils from reputable sources.

9. **Heat and sunlight destroy essential oils over time.** Don't store your essential oils near a heat source or in direct sunlight, as repeated exposure to heat and sunlight cause deterioration. Keep them somewhere dark and relatively cool, such as inside a box that is in turn stored in a closet.

10. **Essential oils generally retain potency for five years or longer.** When stored in a cool, dark place, essential oils retain potency for five to ten years on average. Citrus oils are the exception; these retain full potency for a maximum of two years.

11. **Dark-colored glass bottles are best.** Most manufacturers package their essential oils in dark-colored amber or sometimes blue glass bottles. When creating essential oil blends, making massage oil, or concocting another recipe that will be stored for more than a few days, package the resulting product in a dark-colored glass bottle to prevent long-term exposure to any type of light. Glass is preferable to metal, as it will not react with the oils, and glazed ceramic containers will also work. Do not use plastic bottles; the essential oils will break down the plastic, sullying your essential oil and potentially creating a mess.

12. **Save by starting small.** You might be tempted to rush out and purchase an entire apothecary's worth of essential oils, but doing so represents quite an investment. Save money and avoid becoming overwhelmed by selecting a few of the most versatile essential oils at first, then work your way toward expanding your inventory. Some of the best essential oils to start with are lavender, lemon, peppermint, rose geranium, rosemary, orange, and tea tree.

13. **Because they are natural, essential oils cannot be patented.** Since essential oils are so effective, you may wonder why they are not part of mainstream medicine. The answer is simple: Pharmaceutical companies cannot patent essential oils, and because drug companies cannot make large profits from them, essential oils are not extensively studied in mainstream laboratories. The majority of what is known about essential oils comes from information passed down over thousands of years of experimentation and personal use, so your doctor is not likely to recommend a natural essential oil therapy over a pharmaceutical one.

14. **Opinions concerning the recommended use of essential oils vary.** Most essential oils can be used without reservation, a few are clearly unsafe, and some are hotly debated, even among professionals belonging to the same organization. If you feel uncomfortable or unsure about how or when to use an essential oil, conduct as much research as possible before determining whether that oil has a place in your self-care plan, or find another essential oil with similar healing benefits that you feel comfortable using.

15. **Apply essential oils as soon as symptoms arise or an injury occurs.** If no improvement is noticed within three to four hours, try a different oil or blend, as every individual is biologically unique. Prominent naturopath Dr. Scott A. Johnson advises multiple methods of application be used to increase efficacy.

THE SCIENCE OF SCENTS
How Aromatherapy Works

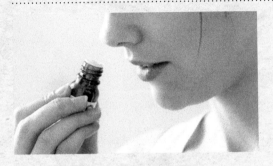

Imagine inhaling the fragrance of a rose in full bloom on a warm summer day, or catching the scent of fresh garlic and rosemary in the kitchen, and consider how those scents bring about a shift in your state of mind. Essential oils, which contain massive concentrations of powerful plant chemicals, stimulate the subconscious with their scents, bringing feelings of alertness, happiness, calm, relaxation, or sleepiness.

Aromatherapy not only has a positive effect on the psyche and spirit by working in concert with the limbic system but it also aids in physical healing. This occurs in two ways:

1. Minuscule essential oil molecules are absorbed into the bloodstream via the lungs when inhaled.
2. These tiny molecules can be absorbed directly into the bloodstream via the skin when added to bathwater, used in body care products, or applied during a massage.

When physically applied to the body, healing essential oils help keep undesirable bacteria and viruses at bay while stimulating the immune system; they also have a powerful detoxifying effect associated with increased lymph and blood flow.

Because of its ability to positively influence emotions, aromatherapy can help mitigate the downward cycle of depression and malaise that often accompanies illness, exhaustion, and periods of prolonged physical or mental stress.

Science has proven time and again that emotional state has the power to change the body's chemistry and that such changes in chemistry directly affect the immune system. By using aromatherapy to keep negative states of being such as stress, tension, and sleeplessness at bay, you can give your overall health a boost. Because of its ability to positively influence the body and mind, aromatherapy is an exceptional form of prevention.

2

GETTING
STARTED WITH
ESSENTIAL OILS

Just as ingredients in medicines can vary, so can the contents of substances labeled as essential oils. Not all essential oils are the same.

While it is easy to get started with essential oils, there are some important things to be aware of before purchasing anything. Often the more research you do, the more potentially confusing information you are likely to encounter concerning quality, source, and which essential oils are best for someone who is just starting out. It is best to determine a select number of essential oils you'd like to start with, and narrow your research to those, at first, to confirm they are right for you.

If you are not sure you will like the aroma of a certain essential oil, consider taking a trip to your local health food store, where it is likely that you will be able to smell samples from different producers. You may also be able to do a patch test while at the store; if this service is offered, consider taking advantage of it.

Essential oils are sold in various quantities, and most have a shelf life of at least one year. It's a good idea to get the smallest size to begin with. Although these tiny bottles don't look like they contain much, you'll be surprised at how long they last. Once you are more familiar with essential oils and know which ones you tend to use quickly, go for a larger bottle. You may save some money by doing so.

Armed with the information in this chapter, you'll find it easy to decipher labels, and it's likely that your shopping experience—for essential oils and the tools needed to work with them—will be targeted and successful.

NOT ALL ESSENTIAL OILS ARE EQUAL

When you read the lists of ingredients in cough syrups, sleep aids, and headache remedies, you'll find artificial flavoring and coloring, high fructose corn syrup, and a plethora of other additives that don't seem like they belong in substances that are meant to bring you better health. Just as ingredients in medicines can vary, so can the contents of substances labeled as essential oils. Not all essential oils are the same.

Perfumeries want consistent fragrances. Leading aromatherapy expert Maria Lis-Balchin warns that the desire for fragrance consistency often leads to adulteration with botanicals or synthetics. Top producers test for adulteration via gas chromatography (sometimes called gas-liquid chromatography) and mass spectroscopy, two separate tests capable of identifying constituents. Labels often carry the abbreviation GC-MS or GLC-MS to indicate that this testing has taken place and the essential oil has been deemed pure.

What You Need to Know Before Purchasing Essential Oils

There are several key factors to keep in mind when shopping for essential oils, each of which is discussed below.

- **Label information** on the bottles of essential oils varies from one company to the next. Unless you are purposefully purchasing a diluted blend or a product containing essential oil as one of its ingredients, the only ingredient listed on the bottle should be the essential oil. Be wary of labels that use the words *perfume oil, fragrance oil,* or *nature identical oil.* These are indicators that the substance in the bottle is probably not 100 percent essential oil.
- **Dark-colored glass bottles** are the standard for essential oils manufacturers. Top manufacturers use cobalt blue, green, violet, and amber bottles, often fitted with orifice reducers rather than droppers, because most droppers allow air to enter the bottle.

- **Look for price variance** in the essential oils offered for sale by the company whose products you are considering. Production costs vary, which means the cost of the essential oils made by a company should also vary. If all the essential oils from a certain company are priced exactly alike, consider them suspect and move on to a different manufacturer's products.

- **A long chain of supply** is a red flag. As you compare essential oils with one another, ask a health food provider or do a little online research to learn about the chain of supply—the producer, wholesaler, mid-level distributor that bottles essential oils for different brands, and the distributor, plus the after-market sources such as online sellers that buy in bulk and resell small quantities of essential oils. The more levels involved, the greater the risk that the essential oils you receive will be adulterated with synthetic fragrances, fillers, bulking agents, and extenders, or have been reconstituted.

- **Folded or concentrated** essential oils produce a stronger scent. These are often best for candles, soaps, household cleaners, and aromatherapy recipes that will be rinsed off or diffused. Rectified or redistilled essential oils are those that have been put through a vacuum once or more to remove impurities; these are perfectly fine for all applications, though you will find that they tend to be costlier than standard essential oils. Certain rectified essential oils are stronger than their counterparts that have been produced using standard techniques, so check specific precautionary information if you are considering using any of these.

- **The choice of whether to buy organics** is up to you. Organic essential oils are grown without herbicides and pesticides, and plants do absorb these substances. There are peripheral considerations regarding the effect that herbicides and pesticides have on the environment. Let your own ideals be your guide.

Get to know organics. There is quite a bit of confusion concerning organic produce and other certified organic products. In the United States, the Department of Agriculture (USDA) holds organic producers to high standards, benefiting the environment and end consumers. Using organic essential oils whenever they are available can reduce your exposure to pesticides, herbicides, and other synthetic substances.

Essential Oil Grades Explained

While some companies market their essential oils with terms such as *aromatherapy grade* or *therapeutic grade*, there is no official grading system for essential oils. These terms vary from one company to the next and are used as a marketing technique. Overlook these labels and focus on other aspects of the essential oil in question:

- Is the company known for quality products?
- Are the essential oils being offered GC-MS tested?
- Are prices in line with similar products offered by other companies? Though there is some pricing variation, most companies price the same type of essential oil within a few dollars. Beware if prices seem extraordinarily low.
- Is there other label information, such as the plant's Latin name and common name?

CHOOSING WHICH TYPE OF ESSENTIAL OILS TO USE

The essential oils that are best for another person might not be the best for you. For example, if you are allergic to a particular plant, you will most likely be allergic to essential oil made from this plant, as shown in a six-year German study in which those who were allergic to chamomile were also proven to be allergic to chamomile essential oil.

There are hundreds of essential oils to choose from. As you decide which essential oils to purchase first, keep the following points in mind:

- Determine which ailments you want to treat, and look for essential oils that are effective in treating these ailments.
- If there is a specific recipe you plan to use, gather all the ingredients.
- If the essential oils are for a baby or young child, be sure to select those that are suitable and safe.
- Consider whether you want to use essential oils for first aid, and choose one or two that will suit your purposes.

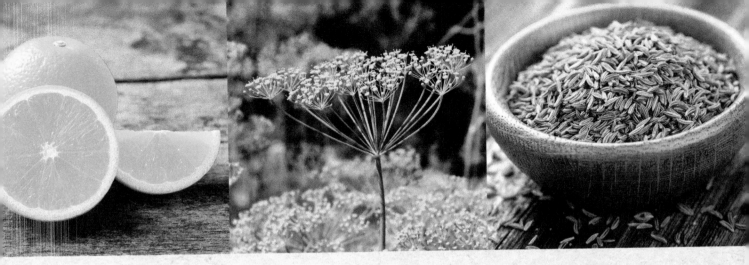

PHOTOSENSITIZING PLANTS
Keep Your Skin Safe

According to Dr. Jillian Stansbury, citrus species aren't the only plants that can lead to phototoxicity. There are many other useful plants that can contribute to sun sensitivity and subsequent damage when consumed or used within 12 hours of sun exposure. Some of these find their way into essential oils, while others might be ingested during a meal or snack.

- Angelica
- Anise
- Bergamot
- Celery
- Cumin
- Dill
- Ginger
- Grapefruit
- Lemon
- Lemon verbena
- Lime
- Mandarin orange
- Orange
- Parsnips
- Tagetes
- Tangerine
- Yuzu

TOOLS AND EQUIPMENT

When working with essential oils, it's vital that you use appropriate tools and equipment. These will help ensure that you get the most from your investment, plus they will help prevent undesirable reactions such as those that occur between essential oils and plastic. The tools and equipment fall under two categories: indispensable and nice to have.

Indispensable

- **Dark-colored glass containers.** Dark-colored glass containers are available in a variety of shapes and sizes, ranging from a single dram to several ounces. Using glass (rather than plastic or metal) ensures that the essential oils do not react with their containers, spoiling the entire contents. Also, using dark-colored glass prevents sunlight from deteriorating the essential oils. These containers are crucial if you plan to make any of your own blends or purchase large quantities of certain oils and store them in smaller bottles inside first aid kits.
- **Glass bowls.** Glass bowls such as those made for food preparation are ideal for preparing aromatherapy products. It's fine to use the ones you may already have in your kitchen; be sure they are perfectly clean before using them with essential oils. Wood, plastic, and metal bowls should be avoided.
- **Glass droppers.** It's very difficult to clean essential oil residue from the inside of a plastic dropper, which is why glass ones are superior to plastic. These are necessary for measuring oils for blends and recipes. Clean them thoroughly after each use, and consider assigning each type of essential oil its own dropper.
- **Labels.** Labels are essential for preventing mix-ups. If you don't want to spring for specially designed essential oil labels, you can use something as simple as masking tape and a permanent marker to differentiate the blends you create from one another.

Nice to Have

- **Dark-colored plastic containers.** These containers are ideal for storing diluted homemade recipes such as shampoo, conditioner, room spray, and many cleaning products. Since the essential oils in most of these recipes are extremely diluted, your preparations won't interact with the plastic containers. These containers also give homemade products an appealing look and are nice for gift giving.

- **Diffuser.** A diffuser distributes a consistent spray of essential oils. These small, quiet appliances are a handy tool in any aromatherapy kit.

- **Glass mixing rods.** Designed for mixing chemicals and other substances that react with metal or plastic, these slender rods are useful for combining essential oils and for stirring recipes containing large quantities of essential oil. A metal spoon, fork, or whisk may be used, if needed, but plastic utensils ought to be avoided.

- **Notebook.** It is a good idea to designate a small notebook or journal for keeping track of basic information about the essential oils you use and how they affect you and your family. You can also use it for making notes about blends you create and for making treatment notes. This doesn't have to be fancy—an inexpensive spiral notebook will work perfectly.

- **Pendant.** One of the easiest ways to enjoy the benefits of essential oil inhalation is with an aromatherapy pendant. They are available in a number of styles, colors, and configurations to suit your taste. Different pendants use different amounts of essential oil, so be sure to follow the instructions that come with the pendant. Pendants and pendant kits are available online and in some health food stores.

- **Small funnels.** Tiny funnels measuring about two inches across at their widest points are typically offered for laboratory use, but as they're ideal for use with essential oils, you'll find them for sale at sites offering aromatherapy tools. They are convenient when pouring oils from one bottle to another to prevent waste. If you decide to purchase inexpensive plastic funnels rather than more costly glass ones, be sure to clean them thoroughly after each use to prevent essential oil residue from eating the plastic.

- **Storage box.** A sturdy, padded storage box is ideal for insulating your essential oils, preventing breakage, and preventing light from penetrating essential oil bottles. This can be something as simple as a small bin lined with a few tea towels, or as elaborate as one of the specially constructed boxes available for sale on an aromatherapy site. While it's not necessary to store your oils in a box, particularly when you're just starting out, doing so will keep you organized while protecting your investment.

STORING TIPS AND INSTRUCTIONS

Although essential oils will not turn rancid as oils containing fatty acids will, they do deteriorate and oxidize, losing their therapeutic properties over time. By storing your essential oils properly, you will prevent premature deterioration.

- **Store essential oils in glass bottles.** Because essential oils are volatile, they will often react with plastic, causing contamination.
- **Keep your essential oils cool.** Exposure to heat causes essential oils to deteriorate rapidly. According to prominent aromatherapy expert Robert Tisserand, essential oils that are kept in the refrigerator last as much as twice as long as those kept at room temperature. Allow refrigerated essential oils to come to room temperature before using them.
- **Prevent exposure to light.** Light also causes essential oils to deteriorate, with sunlight being the worst offender due to its warmth.
- **Do not leave droppers in essential oil bottles.** Even glass droppers allow small amounts of air to enter essential oil bottles, exposing them to contaminants and causing them to deteriorate. Plastic droppers sometimes dissolve in the essential oil when left in place, ruining the whole bottle. Use screw-top caps.
- **Cap oils tightly when not in use.** Because of their volatility, essential oils evaporate rapidly if not capped tightly between uses.
- **Store carrier oils in the refrigerator.** Carrier oils are delicate and can go rancid within a few months if exposed to heat. Keep them refrigerated when not in use and allow them to come to room temperature between eight and twelve hours before use.

- **Keep essential oils away from open flames.** Essential oils are highly flammable and should be stored away from open flames.
- **Be aware of each essential oil's shelf life.** Check the shelf life for each essential oil you purchase and use it accordingly. Some oils retain potency for as little as six months, while others remain fully potent for years. Noted aromatherapist K. G. Stiles warns that when essential oils begin to thicken, smell more acidic, or take on a cloudy appearance, they are beginning to oxidize.

WHAT ARE CARRIER OILS?

Sometimes referred to as fixed oils or natural base oils, carrier oils are used for diluting essential oils prior to application. Most are made with vegetables, nuts, or seeds, and all are excellent for creating natural massage oils that nourish and moisturize the skin while imparting an essential oil's specific benefits.

- **Almond oil:** Often labeled as sweet almond oil, almond oil has a light, faintly sweet aroma and a faint yellow hue. Rich in vitamins B_2, B_6, and E, it is popular for use in commercially prepared lotions, creams, and massage oils. It is suitable for sensitive skin, but it is not a good choice for anyone with allergies to tree nuts. If considering using it for a baby or young child not previously exposed to almonds, conduct a patch test by placing a single drop of almond oil on the child's arm and waiting 24 hours for signs of an adverse reaction.
- **Aloe vera oil:** A fast-penetrating moisturizer, aloe vera oil is made with a base oil and macerated aloe. Offering the healing power of aloe, this carrier oil is popular for use in preparations meant for wounds or burns. While aloe vera gel and aloe vera juice are widely available, aloe vera oil may prove difficult to find in some areas.

Use aloe to speed healing, unless you are allergic to latex. According to the University of Maryland Medical Center, aloe vera has been widely studied and has been proven beneficial in speeding the healing process. Because of its natural latex content, it is not recommended for anyone with a latex allergy.

- **Avocado oil:** A very rich carrier oil with a sweet, nutty aroma, avocado oil has a thick consistency and a deep, olive green color. It is highly nourishing to skin and hair alike, making it a good addition to body creams and conditioners, but its heavy texture can be off-putting.

- **Calendula oil:** Be sure not to confuse calendula carrier oil with calendula essential oil. This rich oil is made with various vegetable oils that have been infused with calendula blossoms, and typically has a pleasant aroma. Rich in vitamins A, B_1, B_2, and B_6, it is ideal for salves and lotions meant to nourish and heal compromised skin. Not all calendula oils are the same, so conduct some research prior to purchase to ensure the base oil is one that appeals to you. Common base oils include olive oil, sunflower oil, and jojoba oil.

- **Evening primrose oil:** High in fatty acids, including omega-6 essential fatty acids, evening primrose oil is an excellent choice for use in skin care preparations such as those intended for the treatment of eczema. Because it is more costly than most other carrier oils, it is usually blended with less expensive oils before the addition of essential oil.

- **Grape seed oil:** A thin, lightweight oil that imparts a glossy sheen to skin, grape seed oil has a very pale green-yellow tinge and a slightly sweet, nutty aroma. Although this carrier oil is an excellent one for use in massage oils and for general aromatherapy use, it is often solvent extracted, meaning chemical residue may be present. Choose a brand that has been expeller pressed.

- **Hazelnut oil:** Hazelnut oil has a light, sweet, nutty aroma and a pale yellow color. Because it penetrates rapidly, it is a good choice for all-around aromatherapy use and is popular for making massage oil designed for those who suffer from oily skin. If you are looking for a highly moisturizing carrier oil, you may want to select something other than hazelnut oil, as it has a slightly astringent quality.

- **Jojoba oil:** Unique among carrier oils for its thick, waxy feel, jojoba oil has a distinct aroma that most people find pleasant. Highly moisturizing and ideal for massage, it is much more stable than most carrier oils and has an indefinite shelf life. It is an excellent choice for anyone with acne-prone skin, but it should be used conservatively, as applying an excessive amount can lead to shiny, oily-looking skin. If applying it to your face, use just four or five drops at a time.
- **Macadamia oil:** A light yellow color with a sweet, nutty aroma, macadamia oil is thicker than many other carrier oils, making it quite slippery and excellent for formulating massage oils. While its fragrance is appealing, it can be overpowering.
- **Olive oil:** Although olive oil typically costs less than most other carrier oils and has a relatively long shelf life of up to two years, it is among the least favorite oils available. Thick and somewhat greasy, its olive aroma can be overpowering. If you are in a bind, olive oil will work for aromatherapy; just be certain you have chosen a cold-pressed extra-virgin or virgin olive oil.
- **Sesame oil:** A staple in Asian cuisine, sesame oil has a distinct aroma that can be overpowering when used in aromatherapy blends. For this reason, it is typically blended with other carrier oils prior to use. Thick, viscous, and slow to absorb, it is excellent for massage.
- **Walnut oil:** According to Dr. Cathy Wong, walnut oil may aid in treating skin conditions such as psoriasis, warts, and canker sores. As this carrier oil is rich in omega-3 essential fatty acids, it is also an excellent choice for nourishing and replenishing dry, damaged skin. It is not suitable for anyone with a walnut allergy; if you are allergic to other tree nuts, it may cause irritation or an allergic reaction.
- **Wheat germ oil:** With its dark color and strong aroma, wheat germ oil can quickly overpower aromatherapy blends, but its ability to nourish skin makes it a favorite for use in facial moisturizers and body creams. Be sure to choose expeller-pressed wheat germ oil over that which has been solvent extracted, and keep it refrigerated to prevent early spoilage. Even under ideal conditions, wheat germ oil has a shelf life of just about two months.

SAFETY FIRST

Although many essential oils are generally considered safe by the FDA, it is important to take safety into consideration, no matter which of them you decide to use. Each of the essential oil entries found in Chapter Five includes safety information; refer to this section for more in-depth details as needed.

- **Avoid abortifacient essential oils if pregnant.** Abortifacient essential oils are strong emmenagogues that can bring on severe bleeding and abortion. These oils should not be considered as a means to terminate a pregnancy, as they are innately toxic and will cause harm to the pregnant woman. They include:

▪ Mugwort	▪ Sage	▪ Tansy
▪ Parsley seed	▪ Sassafras	▪ Thuja
▪ Pennyroyal	▪ Savin	▪ Wormwood
▪ Rue		

- **Avoid contact with banned essential oils.** Because of toxicity, certain essential oils have been banned by the International Fragrance Association, whose standards, according to their website, "form the basis for the globally accepted and recognized risk management system for the safe use of fragrance ingredients." These essential oils have been shown to contain carcinogens, cause irritation, or lead to excessive sensitization, and are not suitable for aromatherapy use. See the sidebar on Dangerous Plants for a list of banned essential oils (page 43).

- **Cancer patients should use essential oils with care.** If you have cancer, consult your doctor concerning the use of any essential oils, even for massage. Although many of them can be therapeutic, the National Cancer Institute cautions that some essential oils should be avoided by those suffering from cancer. These include:

▪ Aniseed	▪ Clove	▪ Laurel
▪ Basil	▪ Fennel	▪ Nutmeg
▪ Bay	▪ Ho leaf	▪ Star anise
▪ Cinnamon		

If you have an estrogen-dependent form of cancer, avoid contact with the following essential oils, as well:

- Citronella
- Eucalyptus
- Lavender
- Lemongrass
- Verbena

Those who suffer from melanoma and other forms of skin cancer should also avoid contact with citrus essential oils and other essential oils that have sun-sensitizing properties.

- **Keep essential oils out of reach of children.** Although there are numerous essential oils that are safe for children and babies, essential oils should be kept out of reach of children.
- **Use half-strength preparations for children.** With the exception of recipes formulated specifically for babies or children, assume all other recipes are formulated for adults. These recipes should be prepared at half their strength for use on anyone under age 12.
- **Use caution when administering steam inhalation treatments to children.** Steam inhalations for those age 12 and older are typically meant to last until the solution cools, though some call for shorter treatment periods. When administering a steam inhalation treatment to anyone younger than 12 years old, keep treatments to one minute per session, and do not leave the child unattended.
- **Take care when using essential oils for seniors.** Elderly, frail, and bedridden people are often more sensitive to essential oils than are average adults. Consider formulating treatments at half their strength to prevent skin irritation or sensitization.
- **Avoid emmenagogue essential oils during pregnancy.** While emmenagogues do not have abortifacient qualities, they do stimulate menses and should be avoided by women who are pregnant. These include:

- Angelica
- Cinnamon
- Clary sage
- Fennel
- German chamomile
- Ginger
- Jasmine
- Juniper
- Marjoram
- Myrrh
- Nutmeg
- Peppermint
- Roman chamomile
- Rose
- Rosemary

- **Some essential oils may cause drowsiness.** While this is a wonderful quality for those suffering from sleeplessness, it is important to avoid certain essential oils when driving, operating machinery, or concentrating on other important tasks. Essential oils that cause drowsiness include:

  - Benzoin
  - Carnation
  - Clary sage
  - Geranium
  - German chamomile
  - Hops
  - Hyacinth
  - Lavender
  - Linden
  - Mace
  - Marjoram
  - Neroli
  - Nutmeg
  - Ormenis flower
  - Petitgrain
  - Roman chamomile
  - Sandalwood
  - Spikenard
  - Valerian
  - Vetiver
  - Ylang-ylang

- **Use caution if suffering from hypertension or cardiac disease.** There are some essential oils that can calm and relax you, while others may cause a harmful increase in blood pressure or lead to heart palpitations. Research any essential oils you are considering before trying them.

- **If you decide to use essential oils internally, ensure you take only those that are not linked to liver toxicity.** While this book does not recommend ingesting essential oils, after proper research, you may decide it is right for you. However, many essential oils that are suitable for external use are not suitable for therapeutic ingestion. These include the banned essential oils (page 43) and the following:

  - Aniseed
  - Basil
  - Bay
  - Buchu
  - Cassia
  - Cinnamon
  - Clove
  - Fennel
  - Tarragon

Practice sun safety. Many essential oils are photosensitizing, meaning they can cause skin to be more sensitive to the sun or any other source of ultraviolet light. Sunburns and skin damage happen faster and more easily when photosensitizing essential oils are present, so use these at least 12 hours before planned exposure. See page 33 for a complete list of photosensitizing essential oils.

DANGEROUS PLANTS
Essential Oils to Avoid

The planet is teeming with plants, both beneficial and dangerous. While the following is by no means a complete list of the world's toxic plants, it contains those that are sometimes formulated into essential oils and offered for sale, often by unscrupulous dealers. These should be neither ingested nor applied topically, even when heavily diluted.

- **Bitter almond**—contains cyanide
- **Boldo**—causes convulsions
- **Cade oil crude***—carcinogenic
- **Camphor**—may be inhaled; can cause toxicity if ingested
- **Cassia**—irritates mucus membrane and can cause severe skin rash
- **Costus root***—sensitizer
- **Elecampane***—sensitizer
- **Fig leaf absolute***—sensitizer
- **Horseradish***—irritates mucus membranes, eyes, and skin
- **Jaborandi leaf***—toxic
- **Mustard***—irritates mucus membranes, eyes, and skin; toxic

- **Nightshade***—toxic
- **Non-distilled Peru balsam***—sensitizer
- **Pennyroyal***—causes acute liver and lung damage; abortifacient
- **Rue***—abortifacient, irritant, neuro-toxin, toxic
- **Sassafras***—carcinogenic, can be lethal
- **Savin***—abortifacient, sensitizer, skin irritant, toxic
- **Southernwood***—toxic
- **Stinging nettle***—toxic
- **Stryax gum***—sensitizer
- **Tansy**—contains high levels of the poison thujone; causes convulsion, uterine bleeding, organ failure, respiratory arrest, and death
- **Tea absolute***—sensitizer
- **Thuja**—abortifacient, neurotoxin, poison
- **Verbena***—sensitizer
- **Wormseed***—causes liver and kidney toxicity; neurotoxin
- **Wormwood***—contains the poison thujone; abortifacient, causes convulsions, leads to unpleasant hallucinations, neurotoxin

*Indicates banned oil

3

ESSENTIAL OIL
APPLICATION
METHODS

The manner in which you apply essential oils has a direct effect on the way they impact your body and mind.

Essential oils can enhance your daily life in a plethora of ways. The same essential oils you rely on for first aid can often be used to improve your indoor environment by freshening air naturally. In addition, they often prove useful for treating minor illnesses, and can be added to body care products such as lotion, shampoo, and conditioner.

The manner in which you apply essential oils has a direct effect on the way they impact your body and mind. If, for example, you are using lavender essential oil to promote restful sleep, you may use it in a bath, apply it in a balm, diffuse some in your bedroom as you are falling asleep, or try several methods in combination to enhance efficacy. If you are using that same lavender essential oil to speed healing, you might formulate a synergistic essential oil blend or salve to keep on hand for minor burns and wounds, or you might just apply a simpler formula made with a few drops of lavender essential oil blended with a small amount of your favorite carrier oil.

Essential oils are most often used topically or inhaled. Topical application is typically combined with inhalation by default. For example, when you use an essential oil as part of a massage oil, you benefit from absorption as well as from inhalation.

Many of the essential oils listed in Chapter Four may be used for a variety of purposes. This chapter contains detailed information about application methods as well as guidelines for the safe, effective use of each method.

AROMATIC

Aromatic methods of essential oil application are those in which single essential oils or blends are inhaled in some way. Some methods expose your body to more essential oil than others; choose the one that best meets your needs, whether you hope to relax, concentrate better, or accomplish some other goal.

Diffuse rosemary essential oil to enhance memory. A team of psychologists at England's Northumbria University conducted a series of tests, proving that inhaling rosemary essential oil enhanced memory functions. Diffuse this appealing essential oil while working or studying to reap the benefits.

Diffusion

One of the simplest, most popular methods of aromatic essential oil application is diffusion. There are many different types of diffusers on the market, and not all are created equal.

- *Guidelines:* To get the most from diffused essential oils, choose a cold-air diffuser that uses ultrasonic vibrations to break the oils up into a fine mist, which remains suspended in the air for hours, freshening while treating you to the therapeutic properties of the essential oil of your choice. Be sure to follow the manufacturer's directions for the amount and use of an essential oil.
- *Benefits:* Once suspended in air, an essential oil's aroma helps enhance a room's atmosphere while simultaneously providing you with its specific physical or emotional benefits. If you're hoping to create cheerful, harmonious feelings, for example, tangerine or lemon essential oil will help you do so. If you are hoping to clear airborne pathogens, diffusing eucalyptus essential oil or an antibacterial blend will prove effective.

Essential oils don't simply mask odors as many commercially produced chemical air fresheners do; instead, they interact with the molecules that our bodies interpret as odors. Even if you have no specific emotional or health need, consider diffusing essential oils in your home or work environment on a regular basis. Doing so will, at the very least, relax your mind, alleviate tension, and make indoor air more enjoyable to breathe.

■ **Safety:** Always follow the manufacturer's instructions when using a diffuser. Most warn against using water, vegetable oil, commercially formulated massage oil, or overly thick, undiluted essential oils, as these may clog or damage the diffuser. Finally, you should never diffuse clove or cinnamon essential oils unless they are part of a blend specifically indicated for diffusion. These powerful, spice-based essential oils contain compounds capable of burning the nasal membranes if micro-mist is inhaled.

Direct Inhalation

Certain essential oils are suitable for direct inhalation, which is a powerfully effective yet simple method for obtaining the many benefits of aromatherapy.

■ **Guidelines:** Direct inhalation is easy to do. Begin by placing a few drops of a single essential oil or blend in the palm of your hand, then rub your hands together. Cup them over your nose and mouth, and inhale deeply. Take three to five deep breaths, then relax for at least three minutes before continuing with your day.
If you are not comfortable with applying essential oils directly to your hands but want to enjoy the benefits of direct inhalation, you can simply cup your hands around the bottle and take three to five deep breaths. Cap the bottle before taking a few minutes to relax.

■ **Benefits:** Direct inhalation offers close-up exposure to an essential oil's volatile molecules, allowing you to experience its effects immediately. Benefits vary from one essential oil to the next; these may include a positive influence on emotion, improved learning, reduced appetite, improvement in certain bodily functions, and more.

- **Safety:** Ensure that you check an essential oil's profile before direct inhalation, as some essential oils are not suitable for use with this method of application. Do not allow essential oils to come into contact with the eyes during direct inhalation.

Hot Water Vapors

If you are suffering from a cold, allergies, or other ailment that affects the upper respiratory system, you may want to try a remedy that calls for topping a bowl of steaming hot water with a few drops of essential oil. These treatments are simple, effective, and inexpensive.

Beat respiratory problems with essential oils. Dr. Joie Power recommends inhaling essential oils to combat respiratory illness, as this method brings the essential oils into contact with respiratory tract tissues. Eucalyptus, lemon, rosemary, and tea tree essential oils are a few to try.

- **Guidelines:** Using hot water vapors to deliver essential oils to your respiratory system is simple. Procure a bowl, the essential oil of your choice, a towel to place beneath the bowl to catch any drips, and a towel large enough to drape over your head, shoulders, and the bowl. After placing the first towel on the table, set the bowl on top of it. Pour steaming hot water into the bowl and add three to five drops of essential oil. Sitting comfortably in front of the bowl, drape the second towel over your head, shoulders, and the bowl. With your eyes closed, breathe the vapors for at least one minute or until the steam subsides, if preferred. Emerge from the towel for fresh air as needed.
  It is advisable that you keep a box of tissues close at hand during this treatment, as it encourages sinus drainage. Blow your nose as needed throughout the process.
- **Benefits:** When delivered to the respiratory system via steam, certain essential oils aid in relieving congestion and decreasing mucus membrane inflammation. Sore throat, blocked sinuses, irritation, and dryness are also alleviated during the process of inhaling essential oils and hot water vapors.

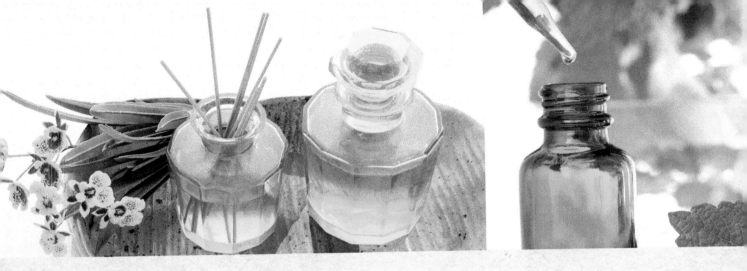

HOW TO DIFFUSE

Essential oil diffusers are versatile and easy to use. While you'll want to follow the instructions that accompany your diffuser, you'll find this step-by-step guide useful as you venture deeper into the world of aromatherapy.

1. Read the instructions that accompany your diffuser, and familiarize yourself with its parts.
2. Add the required amount of essential oil to the diffuser.
3. Decide on a location for the diffuser. A high shelf or mantle might be the ideal place to set the diffuser; this will allow for wide distribution of the essential oil while keeping it out of reach of small children or curious pets.
4. Activate the diffuser.
5. Enjoy the aromatherapy benefits of the essential oil you have chosen. You may want to meditate, relax with your eyes closed, or listen to some music while breathing deeply and regularly.
6. Once finished with the diffusion process, clean your diffuser following the manufacturer's recommendations.
7. Store the diffuser when it's not being used. This will keep it clean while preventing accidental damage.

- **Safety:** Emerge from the towel for fresh air as needed. If you feel that the water vapors are too hot, allow the water to cool somewhat before continuing. If you begin to feel lightheaded or nauseous while using this remedy, stop immediately. Keep your eyes closed while breathing the vapors, as the essential oil in the steam may irritate your eyes.

  Children younger than 12 years old may use this method for up to one minute per treatment. Never leave a child unattended while administering this remedy.

Humidifier or Vaporizer

If you don't have a diffuser, consider using a humidifier to disperse essential oil throughout your living or work space.

- **Guidelines:** To effectively use essential oils with a humidifier, place several drops of the oil of your choice on a tissue or cloth. Place this in front of the humidifier's air intake so the essential oil's molecules blend with the water vapor being emitted.
- **Benefits:** Humidifiers and vaporizers can be used throughout your home to make air more comfortable to breathe, particularly during the winter months. Some people enjoy the background noise of these machines, and others find they help soothe allergy and sinus symptoms. Adding essential oils scents the air while exposing those who breathe it to the specific benefit of the essential oil being used.
- **Safety:** Do not use cinnamon or clove essential oils with a humidifier or vaporizer, as these oils can burn the mucus membranes lining the nasal passages, sinuses, and airway.

  Some sources advise users to put essential oils directly into vaporizers or humidifiers. This is a less effective method of dispersal, and prolonged use of essential oils can cause the machines' plastic parts to become sticky or degrade.

Indirect Inhalation

Any method of inhaling essential oils other than direct inhalation is a form of indirect inhalation. Some examples include diffusion, water vapors, or even just putting a few drops of essential oil on a cotton ball and placing it near your laptop's exhaust fan.

Relax with an essential oil massage. Massage is among the most beneficial ways to experience indirect inhalation. A 2013 study conducted at Korea's Eulji University Hospital concluded that high blood pressure sufferers who received massages with essential oils experienced significant reduction in blood pressure along with improved sleep quality.

- **Guidelines:** When choosing an indirect inhalation method, select the one that works best for the situation at hand. Try different methods to see which you prefer.
- **Benefits:** With indirect inhalation, you enjoy fresher indoor air along with enhanced feelings of overall well-being. You may also experience some therapeutic effects of the essential oil you have chosen to use. Sensitive individuals may find that indirect inhalation methods suit them better than direct inhalation.
- **Safety:** Follow instructions carefully after choosing an indirect inhalation method. Ensure that you keep all essential oils and equipment out of reach of young children.

Vent or Fan

Because vents and fans promote air circulation, they are ideal for dispersing essential oils throughout large spaces.

- **Guidelines:** Using essential oils with a vent or fan is very easy—simply place several drops of essential oil on a cotton ball, then put the cotton ball in close proximity to the vent or fan of your choice.

- ***Benefits:*** Vents and fans can be found in all kinds of places, including homes, offices, cars, and hotel rooms. You can enjoy the benefits that accompany the indirect inhalation of the essential oil of your choice anywhere, so long as you have a few basic, portable supplies with you.
- ***Safety:*** It's a good idea to set the cotton ball on a small glass or ceramic saucer to prevent the essential oil from coming into contact with surfaces that could be adversely affected. Be sure to keep cotton balls and other items used with vents and fans out of reach of children and pets.

Internal

Essential oils may seem innocuous, but they are extremely potent. Keeping in mind that a single drop of essential oil contains the therapeutic power of a much larger number of plants, it is vital that you understand the potential harm that could result from ingesting essential oil without first consulting a doctor who is familiar with using it safely.

It is true that small amounts of essential oil can be used in culinary applications, and it is also true that the French method of aromatherapy calls for the ingestion of carefully prepared compounds containing essential oils. When used internally, essential oils must be taken with great care, and physician oversight is highly recommended. The amounts typically prescribed for internal use are minuscule—usually between one and three drops per dose depending on the illness, the essential oil, and the patient's personal profile. Most of these protocols recommend that essential oils be ingested for short periods only, discouraging prolonged use.

Essential oils are typically diluted with warm water, soy milk, or rice milk prior to ingestion when prescribed for oral use, as certain oils such as oregano and cinnamon can cause stinging or burning and potentially cause damage to the mouth and esophagus.

Potential side effects of ingestion include poisoning caused by an overdose or adulteration, along with a stinging sensation in the mouth, indigestion or an upset stomach, and diarrhea. Stomach pain, chest pain, severe nausea, and grogginess might also occur.

It is vital that you be aware of the potential problems that ingesting specific essential oils could cause, and to seek the advice of a qualified health care professional who can determine whether the ingestion of essential oils is appropriate for you.

For safety reasons, this book does not include any remedies that involve ingesting essential oils.

TOPICAL

Applying essential oils and products containing essential oils to your skin allows them to quickly enter the bloodstream and rapidly circulate throughout the body. Indirect inhalation typically accompanies topical application, offering an additional benefit. Depending on the reason for using an essential oil, you may apply an essential oil remedy to the affected site or you may apply essential oils to certain pressure points or reflexology points.

Acupressure

Acupressure involves the application of direct pressure to specific points on the body. Intended to aid in pain relief, help eliminate headaches, stop nausea, and alleviate other problems, it is part of Chinese medicine. Although typically accomplished with pressure alone, acupressure is sometimes enhanced by the addition of essential oils.

- *Guidelines:* Acupressure is also referred to as acupuncture without needles, and at least a basic knowledge of the body's meridians is necessary for successful treatment. Beginners can easily learn which pressure points to use to encourage relaxation, release tension, and stimulate healing. When choosing essential oils for use in acupressure, be certain to select those that are suitable for addressing the problem at hand.
- *Benefits:* When combining essential oils and acupressure, you benefit not just from the properties of the essential oil you choose but also from the correct application of the chosen acupressure techniques.

■ **Safety:** While acupressure is a simple, straightforward process, it's vital that you learn how to use it appropriately before implementing treatments. The body's underlying structures are delicate and can be easily damaged, so err on the side of caution when considering treatment options.

Acupuncture

Acupuncture is the practice of inserting specialized needles into specific points along the body's meridians, after which they are sometimes manipulated manually or via electrical stimulation. Only a certified acupuncturist should employ this method of treatment.

■ **Guidelines:** Seek an acupuncturist who is willing to use essential oils during therapy. While some professionals avoid the use of essential oils, others use them extensively.
■ **Benefits:** The benefits of acupuncture are numerous; it is used to treat a vast array of health conditions, ranging from chronic pain to infertility. When an acupuncturist chooses essential oils to incorporate into treatment, he or she selects those most likely to enhance health and well-being based on the condition or symptoms presented by the patient.
■ **Safety:** While most acupuncturists are certified, some individuals practice without certification. Seek a qualified acupuncturist and ensure that he or she uses appropriate sterilization techniques.

Bath

Essential oils add fragrance to baths while treating the body and mind to the unique benefits they imbue. Adding essential oils to your bathtub is one of the simplest, most pleasant ways to use them.

■ **Guidelines:** Just add three to six drops of essential oil or an essential oil blend to your bath while the water is running. This ensures that the oil blends with the water rather than simply floating on top. Soak in the tub for as long as you like and moisturize your skin after getting out.

- **Benefits:** Taking a bath with essential oils is beneficial because the essential oils can easily penetrate the skin, and you receive the secondary benefit of indirect inhalation. The specific benefits vary depending on which essential oil or blend you add to your bathwater, and include relaxation, pain relief, and relief from cold symptoms such as congestion and sinus pressure.
- **Safety:** Essential oils are often added to baths along with a carrier oil, which moisturizes skin during the bathing process. Be careful not to slip when getting in and out of the bathtub.

Cold Packs

Cold packs reduce inflammation caused by strains and sprains, and they're also ideal for cooling off naturally in hot weather. Adding essential oil increases a cold pack's versatility and makes it more pleasurable to use.

- **Guidelines:** Cold packs can be made of fabric and filled with rice, buckwheat, or another grain that has been mixed with eight to ten drops of the essential oil or blend of your choice. Store packs in the freezer, inside sealed storage bags. Use as needed, refreezing the cold packs after each treatment. You can make cold packs any size you like; just avoid overfilling them to ensure they remain flexible. Periodically dab a few drops of essential oil on the packs to refresh them.
- **Benefits:** Cold packs made with essential oils are ideal for soothing headaches, easing sinus congestion, and relaxing muscle cramps. Select the essential oils you'll be using according to your specific needs.
- **Safety:** Essential oil cold packs are much safer than those containing dry chemicals, and they're not as strong as ice packs. Even so, be sure not to use them over fragile or broken skin, and use caution when applying essential oil cold packs to areas with poor circulation. Keep the cold pack in place for no longer than 20 minutes per treatment.

Compresses

Hot and cold compresses are made with fabric, water, and essential oil. Very simple to prepare, they are ideal for improving circulation, reducing pain, and treating many types of minor injuries, including sprains and strains.

- **Guidelines:** Both hot and cold compresses can be made with approximately a pint of water, four or five drops of essential oil, and a small towel or other piece of absorbent fabric. Compresses can be made with the essential oil added to the water or put directly on the skin and then covered with the compress. In the first method, after mixing the drops in the water, allow the fabric to absorb the water and essential oil, then wring it out, fold to size, and place the compress on top of the affected area. In the second method, which is most often used with the hot compress treatments given in this book, the essential oil is placed or rubbed onto the skin and then covered with the wrung-out fabric.

  With both methods, the compress can be covered with plastic wrap to keep it in place and prevent drips; you may also cover it with another towel or a self-gripping bandage to keep it in place. Leave the compress on until it reaches body temperature.

- **Benefits:** Hot essential oil compresses are ideal for treating pain, including chronic muscle discomfort, rheumatism, menstrual cramps, and toothaches. Cold essential oil compresses are useful for soothing headaches and cooling fevers, and they're also ideal for treating bruises, swelling, sprains, and inflammation.

- **Safety:** Since the essential oil in a compress will be in contact with your skin, use only those oils you've tested or used in the past. Ensure that hot compresses are not so hot that they cause discomfort or burns.

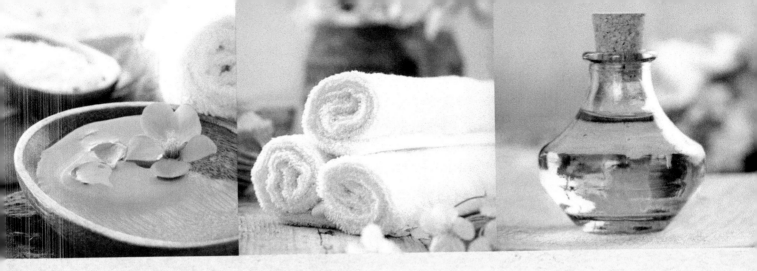

HOW TO MAKE A COMPRESS

Hot and cold compresses are made and used in the same manner, either with the essential oil being placed into the water or applied directly to the skin. For hot compresses, use very hot water (but not so hot that it will burn your skin or cause discomfort). For cold compresses, use extremely cold water that has been kept in the refrigerator or strained through ice in a colander or cocktail shaker.

1 pint hot or iced water
3 to 5 drops essential oil

1. Pour the hot or cold water into a wide-mouth bowl.
2. Add your chosen essential oil to the water or apply it directly to the skin.
3. Fold a hand towel into a compact square with at least three layers.
4. Lay the towel gently on top of the water and allow the towel to absorb as much water as possible.
5. Wring the excess water from the towel back into the bowl.
6. Smooth out the wrinkles in the towel and lay it on top of the affected area.
7. If desired, use a layer of plastic wrap to secure the compress in place. Ensure the plastic wrap completely encases the compress.
8. Apply a self-adhesive bandage over the plastic wrap to keep it in place.
9. Leave the compress on the affected area until it reaches body temperature.
10. Remove the compress and repeat the treatment as many times as necessary for relief.

Direct Application

Applying essential oils or a remedy containing essential oils directly to an affected area is an effective way to manage issues such as cuts, bruises, fungal infections, and other problems that affect the skin as well as pains beneath the skin's surface.

Eliminate tension headaches with peppermint essential oil. A study reported by the University of Maryland Medical Center showed that applying a solution of 10 percent peppermint essential oil to the temples was as effective at relieving tension headaches as acetaminophen. Dilute one drop of peppermint essential oil with nine drops of carrier oil and massage the blend into the temples for quick relief.

- **Guidelines:** Direct application is ideal for situations in which pain relief or antibacterial protection is required. Essential oils blended in carrier oil, pure or neat essential oils, and sprays, salves, and ointments are the most common remedies for minor injuries, rashes, burns, insect bites, and more.
  When planning which essential oils to include in your first aid kit, conduct patch tests to ensure that specific remedies will help promote healing rather than cause harm.
- **Benefits:** With direct application, essential oils are allowed to penetrate the skin quickly. This is a rapid, effective method for treating a wide array of ailments.
- **Safety:** Conduct a patch test before direct application. It's helpful to test new essential oils as soon as you purchase them so that you'll be able to use them with confidence whenever the need arises.
  Keep essential oils away from eyes and mucus membranes. If such exposure occurs, rinse the affected area with milk to neutralize the oil.
  In most cases, essential oils should not be directly applied to blisters or damaged skin; exceptions include those essential oils that heal and soothe skin. Never apply essential oils directly to second- or third-degree burns.

Layering

Layering essential oils is different from creating a blend. In layering, you apply one essential oil, wait for it to be absorbed, then apply the second oil to the same area. Some treatments call for layering more than two essential oils.

- *Guidelines:* Apply the first essential oil to the area to be treated, using an average of one or two drops. Allow the essential oil to be completely absorbed, then apply the second essential oil on top of the first layer. Wait for it to be absorbed before applying a third essential oil, if using more than two. Continue in this manner.
- *Benefits:* Layering essential oils allows you to treat more than one issue at a time. If you have a sprain with bruising, one essential oil might be used to treat the pain, a second essential oil might be used to address swelling, and a third essential oil might be applied to minimize bruising.
- *Safety:* Ensure that you have conducted a patch test for each of the essential oils you plan to use. Use only one or two drops of each essential oil per treatment.

Massage

Essential oils maximize a massage's healing potential by increasing the calming or energizing effect of the massage technique used. A good carrier oil is indispensable for massage.

- *Guidelines:* Use 12 to 15 drops of an essential oil or essential oil blend per ounce of carrier oil. It's a good idea to make small batches and use them up within a few weeks, as this will ensure efficacy and freshness of the massage oil. Bring your massage oil with you to your therapist, or learn some basic massage techniques with a partner and take turns working on each other.
- *Benefits:* With essential oils, massage becomes more than just a relaxing or energizing method for soothing discomfort and encouraging relaxation. The carrier oil nourishes and softens skin while enabling smooth, even massage strokes, and the essential oil is absorbed into the body.

- *Safety:* Even though essential oils are well diluted during a massage, it's best to ensure that you have conducted a patch test with any essential or carrier oils you plan to incorporate into a massage oil.

Shower

Essential oils can be used in the shower, adding fragrance while providing aromatherapy benefits. Add them to unscented shampoos, conditioners, and body washes, or just place a few drops of the desired essential oil on a washcloth to enhance the aromatherapy experience.

- *Guidelines:* Create pleasant, uniquely scented body washes, shampoos, and conditioners by adding 12 to 15 drops of an essential oil to each ounce of unscented product. There are also many wonderful recipes available for formulating your own natural bath and body products.
  To enhance the effectiveness of the essential oil you have chosen, place three to five drops of an essential oil on a damp washcloth and place that on your chest while in the shower, or place the washcloth on the floor of the shower. The heat of the shower will carry the essential oil's vapors into your respiratory system; breathe deeply while relaxing. When you have finished showering, take a moment to rub your legs, arms, and torso with the washcloth, making gentle circular movements and working your way toward your heart.
- *Benefits:* The benefits of using essential oils in the shower depend greatly upon the oil you use. Eucalyptus essential oil will help clear your sinuses if you are congested; rosemary or spearmint essential oil will help energize you in the morning; lavender essential oil will promote relaxation at bedtime. These are just a few examples: Your options are nearly endless.
- *Safety:* As with all applications, be sure you do not have sensitivity to the essential oils you choose before using them in the shower. Be careful not to slip in the shower when using essential oils blended with a carrier oil.

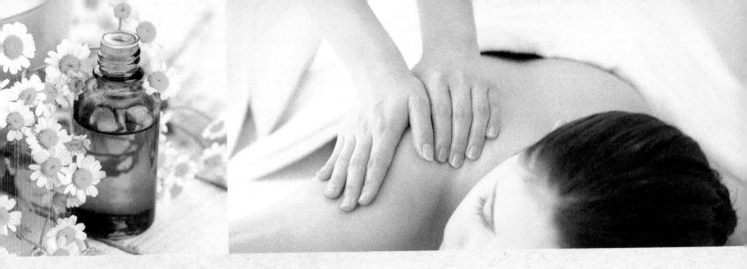

ESSENTIAL MASSAGE TECHNIQUES

There are many massage techniques designed to energize or relax the body. Whether you are massaging your own body or administering a massage to someone else, you'll find that these simple techniques will ensure the massage brings comfort and healing to the recipient.

12 to 15 drops essential oil or blended essential oil
1 ounce carrier oil in a bottle fitted with a lid

1. In a small glass bowl, add the essential oil or blended essential oil and carrier oil, and stir to combine.
2. Set up the massage location. Aim to create a spa-like atmosphere complete with relaxing music. Ensure you are able to move around the area where the massage is being administered.
3. Have the recipient sit or lie comfortably on a sheet.
4. Rub a dime-size amount of massage oil between your hands to warm it.
5. Apply the massage oil to the portion of the recipient's body that requires attention.
6. Give firm enough pressure so you feel the muscle moving under the skin.
7. Using even strokes, massage slowly. When applying pressure, avoid contact with joints and bones.
8. Use additional oil as needed; dry areas such as knees, elbows, and feet often absorb oil quickly.
9. Have the recipient rest comfortably for a few minutes after the massage has come to an end.

4

NATURAL REMEDIES FOR COMMON AILMENTS

Essential oils play an important role in natural healing, making up a major part of Mother Nature's pharmacy.

Minor ailments, cosmetic concerns, and major illnesses can happen to anyone at any time. Instead of running to the drugstore or calling your doctor for non-emergency issues, you have another option. Essential oils play an important role in natural healing, making up a major part of Mother Nature's pharmacy. Many are capable of stopping bacteria, viruses, and fungi, while others work in subtle ways to promote well-being.

Single essential oils aren't like prescription drugs meant for use with just one or two illnesses. Instead, many are capable of working in a variety of ways to treat a wide range of illnesses. In addition, many lend themselves to household use, allowing you to create nontoxic cleansers, insect repellents, and other items that keep the home smelling fresh in a pure, natural way.

In case of serious injury or illness, essential oils should take a back seat to appropriate medical treatment. Injuries such as sprains and strains require immediate first aid, and when severe, may also require a trip to the emergency room. Serious illnesses should be addressed by a physician. If a minor ailment seems to be getting worse rather than improving, seek medical aid. Chronic issues such as arthritis, tendinitis, and rheumatism often respond very well to essential oils, making these natural treatments good substitutes for OTC painkillers that can cause damage to vital organs over time. When used judiciously, essential oils will serve you well.

The following ailments and remedies cover a wide range of topics, from acid reflux to yeast infections. Skim through them at your leisure to familiarize yourself with the subject matter, then refer to individual entries on an as-needed basis. Review the cautions outlined in Chapter Two for those who are pregnant or suffer from a serious or chronic illness and test for sensitivity to the essential oils before using them in a remedy. Also, remember that whenever a remedy advises the use of a dark-colored bottle, be sure to store the remedy in a cool, dark place.

Acid Reflux

Acid reflux occurs when stomach acid moves from the stomach to the esophagus. This happens when a ring of muscle known as the lower esophageal sphincter fails to close completely or opens too often. If acid reflux occurs more than twice weekly, you may have gastroesophageal reflux disease (GERD); see your doctor if this is the case, as severe symptoms could indicate the presence of a hiatal hernia.

ABDOMINAL RUB

MAKES 5 TO 10 TREATMENTS

This remedy relaxes muscles while easing discomfort. If you suffer from frequent acid reflux, a larger batch can be prepared up to two weeks in advance. Those with epilepsy or who are pregnant should avoid this treatment.

2 teaspoons carrier oil
4 drops eucalyptus essential oil
4 drops fennel essential oil
2 drops peppermint essential oil

1. In a dark-colored glass bottle, add the carrier oil along with the eucalyptus, fennel, and peppermint essential oils, and shake well to blend.

2. Using your fingertips, rub several drops of the blend on the upper abdominal area when acid reflux strikes.
3. Repeat this treatment as needed. Store the bottle in a cool, dark place between uses.

Acne

Acne may be mild, moderate, or severe; in all cases, it is caused by sensitivity to androgenic hormones, which are primarily produced during the teenage years. This sensitivity, coupled with the presence of bacteria, dirt, and oil on and beneath the skin, produces blackheads, whiteheads, cysts, bumps, and nodules. Seek medical treatment if acne fails to respond to natural remedies.

GERANIUM SPA FACIAL MASK

MAKES 1 GENEROUS TREATMENT

Geranium essential oil combines with spa facial clay, yogurt, and honey to soothe the inflammation that accompanies acne.

1 tablespoon honey
1 tablespoon plain yogurt
1 tablespoon spa facial clay
6 drops geranium essential oil

1. In a small glass bowl, add the honey, yogurt, clay, and geranium essential oil, and stir to combine.
2. After cleansing the affected areas, use your fingertips to apply the mixture, avoiding the eye area.
3. Leave the mask in place for up to 1 hour, then rinse it off with warm water.
4. Repeat this treatment every 2 to 3 days until symptoms subside.

LAVENDER-TEA TREE ACNE GEL

MAKES 50 TREATMENTS

Geranium, lavender, lemongrass, and tea tree essential oils banish bacteria while soothing inflammation. Use this gel alone or under makeup. This gel will last up to six months.

¼ cup aloe vera gel
10 drops geranium essential oil
10 drops lavender essential oil
6 drops lemongrass essential oil
6 drops tea tree essential oil

1. In a small glass bowl, add the aloe vera gel along with the geranium, lavender, lemongrass, and tea tree essential oils, and stir to combine.
2. Pour the mixture into a wide-mouth, dark-colored glass storage container.
3. Using your fingertips, apply the mixture to the blemishes.
4. Repeat this treatment up to 3 times a day as needed. Store the container in a cool, dark place between uses.

ADD/ADHD

Attention deficit disorder (ADD) and attention deficit hyperactivity disorder (ADHD) are common conditions that affect children, teens, and some adults. Marked by difficulty concentrating, impulsive behavior, and other symptoms, these difficulties respond well to natural remedies and behavior modification. See a doctor if problems worsen or fail to respond to natural treatment.

IMPROVE FOCUS WITH LAVENDER

Lavender essential oil is an excellent remedy for children and adults who suffer from ADD or ADHD, as it addresses anxiety, helps prevent meltdowns, and aids in improving focus and attention. It is also ideal for anyone who has a tendency to become overwhelmed in crowds or stressful situations. Apply 1 drop of lavender essential oil to the sole of each foot before a stressful situation. Repeat this treatment as needed. Here, the essential oil is used neat, but it can be blended with an equal amount of carrier oil prior to application.

CALM WITH LAVENDER AND ROMAN CHAMOMILE

Roman chamomile essential oil is a wonderful antidote to hyperactivity, particularly in children. If you are in a pinch and have just one of these oils, you may use Roman chamomile alone to achieve similar results. Also, an equal amount of lavender and Roman chamomile essential oils may be diffused in the area where the child spends the most time.

2 drops carrier oil
1 drop lavender essential oil
1 drop Roman chamomile essential oil

1. In a small glass bowl, add the carrier oil along with the lavender and Roman chamomile essential oils, and stir to combine.
2. Using your fingertips, apply the blend to the inner wrists or behind the ears.
3. Repeat this treatment once a day as needed.

Addiction Support

Addiction to drugs, alcohol, gambling, and other substances or activities causes serious problems for millions. People who are fighting addiction respond well to natural treatments coupled with behavior modification, intervention, and community support such as a 12-step program. Seek professional help if behaviors surrounding addiction worsen, or if the addict is a threat to himself or herself, or others.

CURB CRAVINGS WITH PEPPERMINT

Peppermint essential oil aids in eliminating the cravings that can lead to a relapse. It can be diffused, worn in an aromatherapy pendant, or simply dotted onto a cotton ball near the person in need of support. Cilantro and grapefruit essential oils also help stop harmful cravings, whether for sugar, alcohol, or other addictive substances.

EASE WITHDRAWAL WITH SANDALWOOD

Withdrawal symptoms cause discomfort and severe anxiety. Sandalwood essential oil has a potent calming effect that can ease the transition from addiction to sobriety. Diffuse the essential oil in the area where the sufferer spends the most time, or add sandalwood essential oil to an aromatherapy pendant. You can also add 1 or 2 drops to a cotton ball in a bath or shower. Grapefruit, lavender, lemon, Roman chamomile, and tangerine essential oils can be used if sandalwood essential oil is not available.

Aging Skin

With aging skin comes a loss of elasticity, plus changes in skin color and texture. Sensitivity often increases, as does dryness. Keeping skin moisturized, preventing excess sun exposure, and eating a healthy diet go a long way toward keeping skin looking its best as you age. See a dermatologist if signs of skin cancer, including multicolor moles or moles larger in diameter than the end of a pencil eraser, are present.

CYPRESS UNDER-EYE THERAPY

MAKES 1 TREATMENT

Cypress essential oil's strong astringent quality makes it ideal for reducing the bags and dark circles that tend to appear beneath the eyes.

2 drops coconut carrier oil
2 drops cypress essential oil (other choices: frankincense, geranium, myrrh, and sandalwood)

1. In a small bowl or in the palm of your hand, add the coconut carrier oil and cypress essential oil.
2. After cleansing the under-eye area, use a cotton ball or your fingertip to gently apply the mixture.
3. Repeat this treatment once a day at bedtime until symptoms subside.

JASMINE-GERANIUM SERUM

MAKES 30 TO 40 TREATMENTS

Jasmine and geranium essential oils balance skin, promoting smoothness while diminishing the appearance of wrinkles. This serum may be stored for up to one year.

1 ounce argan carrier oil
30 drops geranium essential oil
30 drops jasmine essential oil

1. In a dark-colored glass bottle fitted with an orifice reducer, add the argan carrier oil along with the geranium and jasmine essential oils, and shake to blend.
2. Using a cotton pad or your fingertips, apply the blend to the facial area, neck, and décolletage. Use just enough of the blend so the skin absorbs the serum.
3. Repeat the treatment once a day at bedtime. Store the bottle in a cool, dark place between uses.

Allergies

Red eyes, sneezing, a runny nose, itchiness, and even hives, eczema, and asthma attacks can accompany allergies. Seasonal allergies, including allergies to various molds and pollens, happen all throughout the year for some sufferers, and pet allergies can happen at home or when a sufferer comes into contact with domestic animals such as dogs, cats, and horses. Seek professional help if natural allergy remedies do not work for you.

LEMON-MINT MIST

MAKES 20 TO 30 TREATMENTS

Lavender, lemon, and peppermint essential oils ease inflammation while bolstering the immune system to make allergies less problematic. This mist has an appealing fragrance and may be used several times daily.

4 ounces purified water
30 drops lavender essential oil
30 drops lemon essential oil
30 drops peppermint essential oil

1. In a dark-colored glass spray bottle, add the water along with the lavender, lemon, and peppermint essential oils, and shake well to blend.
2. Spray this blend throughout any indoor spaces where allergy sufferers spend time.
3. Repeat this treatment as needed. Shake the bottle before each use.

NASAL ALLERGY IRRIGATION

MAKES 1 TREATMENT

Reduce the inflammation that accompanies severe allergies with this simple, effective treatment. Do not use this with children under 12 years old unless they can tolerate a neti pot.

8 ounces warm purified water
¼ teaspoon fine salt
5 drops lavender essential oil
5 drops lemon essential oil
3 drops peppermint essential oil

1. In a neti pot, add the water and salt.
2. Add the lavender, lemon, and peppermint essential oils to the salt water, and stir to combine.
3. Using the neti pot, perform nasal irrigation, then gently blow the nose.
4. Repeat this treatment up to 3 times a day for relief from allergy symptoms.

Don't fear the neti pot. Neti pots have been used since ancient times to promote clean, healthy sinuses. Today they're available in most drugstores for about $10 or less. Although the concept of flushing the sinuses may sound foreign, this effective treatment is very easy to do. After filling the neti pot, bend over a sink and turn your head to one side. Insert the neti pot's spout into the upper nostril and slowly pour the solution in. Breathe through your mouth and relax as the solution makes its way through your sinuses and out the lower nostril. Switch sides after irrigating the first nostril. Blow your nose gently when finished.

Animal Bites

Animal bites can happen unprovoked, though incitement often precedes bites. Wild animals tend to avoid people but may bite if threatened, cornered, or protecting young. If serious tearing, bone and tendon damage, or very deep puncture wounds are present, seek medical aid. In addition, seek assistance if the potential for rabies exists.

LAVENDER-TEA TREE FLUSH

MAKES 1 TREATMENT

Lavender and tea tree essential oils are well known for their ability to kill bacteria while promoting healing. Brace yourself, because this flush stings quite a bit.

2 ounces hydrogen peroxide
10 drops lavender essential oil
10 drops tea tree essential oil

1. Run cool water over the wound for 1 minute.
2. Pour the hydrogen peroxide onto the affected area.
3. When the fizzing stops, using a dropper, apply the lavender essential oil, then apply the tea tree essential oil. Allow the essential oils to run freely over the wound.
4. Repeat this treatment every 6 to 12 hours for up to 24 hours. Leave the wound open to air in between treatments.

INFECTION PROTECTION

MAKES 20 TO 30 TREATMENTS

Frankincense essential oil helps stop infections while bolstering the immune system, and clove essential oil doubles as a disinfectant and natural pain preventive. This remedy may also be used to treat cuts and scrapes after they have been cleansed.

1 ounce carrier oil
40 drops clove essential oil
40 drops frankincense essential oil

1. In a dark-colored glass bottle fitted with an orifice reducer, add the carrier oil along with the clove and frankincense essential oils, and shake well to blend.
2. Using a dropper, apply the mixture generously to animal bites and other wounds, allowing the essential oil blend to flow freely across the wound.
3. Do not repeat this treatment after a scab has formed.

Anxiety

Fear and anxiety can interfere with daily life. If you often feel nervous, powerless, or worried, it is possible that you are suffering from serious anxiety. Other symptoms include feelings of impending doom, rapid breathing, hyperventilation, trembling, and an increased heart rate. Natural remedies often help sufferers immensely; seek professional help if symptoms do not improve.

STABILIZE WITH VALERIAN

Valerian essential oil is an effective remedy for anxiety, as it aids in stabilizing mood and emotions while relaxing the mind and providing a grounding effect. Diffuse valerian essential oil in the area where you spend the most time or use it in an aromatherapy pendant. You may also dilute the valerian with an equal amount of carrier oil and apply it to your temples.

MELLOW WITH MARJORAM

Marjoram is such a powerful mood stabilizer that it has been nicknamed the "herb of happiness." It calms the nerves while promoting a mellow mindset. In a small bowl, blend marjoram essential oil with an equal amount of a carrier oil before application, or use your fingertips to apply 3 to 5 drops neat to the back of your neck. Enhance marjoram's calming effect by diffusing it, inhaling it directly, or using it with an aromatherapy pendant.

Arthritis

Arthritis symptoms vary depending on the type of arthritis; many sufferers experience joint pain, stiffness, and a debilitating loss of range of motion. While many people with arthritis are past middle age, there are some forms of the disease that strike younger people, including juveniles.

DETOXIFYING ARTHRITIS BATH

MAKES 14 TREATMENTS

Toxins complicate arthritis, and detoxifying essential oils such as cypress, fennel, and juniper can bring rapid relief. Do not use any other arthritis treatments for the two weeks that you use this bath, even those containing essential oils. Do not use this remedy if you have broken skin or are prone to rashes.

30 drops fennel essential oil
16 drops cypress essential oil
10 drops juniper essential oil
2 handfuls Epsom salts
1 handful Dead Sea or rock salt

1. In a dark-colored glass bottle, add the fennel, cypress, and juniper essential oils, and shake well to blend.
2. While the water is running, add the Epsom and Dead Sea salts to the bathtub followed by 4 drops of the essential oil blend.
3. Soak for at least 15 minutes. Use caution when getting out of the bathtub, as it may be slippery.
4. Repeat this treatment once a day for 2 weeks. Store the bottle in a cool, dark place between uses.

SOOTHING PEPPERMINT MASSAGE OIL

MAKES 60 TREATMENTS

Peppermint essential oil alleviates the pain and inflammation that accompanies arthritis. Use this soothing massage oil as often as needed to bring fast relief, naturally.

3½ ounces carrier oil
60 drops peppermint essential oil (other choices: ginger, eucalyptus, or thyme)

1. In a dark-colored glass bottle, add the carrier oil and the peppermint essential oil, and shake well to blend.
2. Allow the massage oil to sit unused for 4 days.
3. Using your fingertips, apply 1 to 3 drops of the blend to each affected area.
4. Repeat this treatment as needed. Store the bottle in a cool, dark place between uses.

Asthma

Asthma is a condition in which narrowed, swollen airways, and the production of excess mucus make breathing difficult. During an asthma attack, a sufferer may experience wheezing, coughing, and shortness of breath, along with tightening of the chest that can lead to panic. Dust mites, mold, pollen, stress, and pet dander are among the most common asthma triggers. See a doctor if natural remedies and trigger avoidance do not prevent symptoms.

LAVENDER STEAM

MAKES 1 TREATMENT

Lavender essential oil relaxes lung spasms and soothes the panic that often accompanies an asthma attack, while steam helps open the airway. Lavender is one of the only essential oils recommended for use during, rather than between, asthma attacks. As always, make sure you are not sensitive to lavender essential oil before relying on this treatment.

3 cups hot water
6 to 8 drops lavender essential oil

1. In a large, shallow bowl, add the hot water and 6 drops of lavender essential oil, and stir to combine.
2. Sit comfortably, tenting your head with a towel over the bowl, and breathe deeply for several minutes, emerging for fresh air as needed.
3. Using your fingertips, apply 1 drop of lavender essential oil to the sole of each foot, and massage it into the skin to intensify the effect while relieving tension.
4. Repeat this treatment once a day as needed.

PREVENTIVE INHALATION RUB

MAKES 30 TREATMENTS

This soothing inhalation rub encourages deep breathing, helping the chest expand; the peppermint essential oil is a strong decongestant that can help prevent asthma attacks. Use this rub between attacks, preferably at bedtime. This remedy is also excellent for soothing cold and flu symptoms.

2 ounces carrier oil
12 drops lavender essential oil
8 drops geranium essential oil
4 drops peppermint essential oil
2 drops marjoram essential oil

1. In a dark-colored glass bottle, add the carrier oil along with the lavender, geranium, peppermint, and marjoram essential oils, and shake well to blend.
2. Using your fingertips, apply a small amount to the chest, and massage it into the skin.
3. Repeat this treatment once a day at bedtime. Store the bottle in a cool, dark place between uses.

Athlete's Foot

Itching, burning, and flaky, yellow, or thickened skin are among the primary symptoms of athlete's foot. Caused by the ringworm fungus, this skin infection is highly contagious. Fortunately, it responds very well to treatment with essential oils. Deep bacterial infections sometimes occur with serious cases of athlete's foot. Seek medical assistance if your symptoms worsen or fail to respond to natural remedies.

ANTIFUNGAL TEA TREE TREATMENT

MAKES 10 TREATMENTS

Tea tree essential oil is a powerful antifungal agent, and it is frequently used to combat athlete's foot. For faster relief, use this remedy as soon as you notice symptoms beginning to develop.

½ ounce carrier oil
30 drops tea tree essential oil

1. In a dark-colored glass bottle, add the carrier oil and tea tree essential oil, and shake well to blend.
2. Using a cotton ball, apply 2 or 3 drops of the blend to the affected area.
3. Repeat this treatment 2 times a day until symptoms subside. Speed the healing process by keeping your feet exposed to open air as often as possible.

Tea tree essential oil kills many viruses, fungi, and bacteria on contact. Numerous studies have proven that tea tree essential oil is effective against a wide range of common viruses, fungi, and bacteria, including the fungus that causes athlete's foot. You can use this remedy with confidence for this and many other common ailments.

SOOTHING CALENDULA-TEA TREE BALM

MAKES 10 TREATMENTS

Use this remedy to heal painful cracks while combating athlete's foot. Tea tree essential oil is the best natural remedy for combating fungus that causes athlete's foot; however, lavender, lemon, or myrrh essential oils can be substituted in a pinch. The calendula carrier oil in this treatment soothes and promotes rapid healing and should not be replaced with an alternate carrier oil.

½ ounce calendula carrier oil, plus 20 to 30 drops
30 drops tea tree essential oil

1. In a dark-colored glass bottle, combine ½ ounce of calendula oil and the tea tree essential oil, and shake well to blend.
2. Using a cotton ball, apply 2 or 3 drops of the blend to the affected area.
3. Using your fingertips, layer 1 to 3 drops of straight calendula oil atop the treatment.
4. Repeat this treatment 2 or 3 times a day until symptoms subside.

Back Pain

Back pain may range from mild to severe, and may happen for a variety of reasons, including strained muscles, slipped vertebrae, trauma, and disease. If back pain worsens, does not respond to natural remedies, or is the result of an accident, you should seek medical assistance as soon as possible. Serious back injuries can lead to complications, including paralysis.

LAVENDER-ROSEMARY SOAK

MAKES 1 TREATMENT

Both lavender and rosemary essential oils promote muscle relaxation, soothing the spasms that often contribute to back pain. Some other essential oils to try in a bath include birch, ginger, and Roman chamomile.

1 teaspoon carrier oil
6 drops lavender essential oil
6 drops rosemary essential oil

1. In a small glass bowl, combine the carrier oil along with the lavender and rosemary essential oils, and stir to combine.
2. Draw a warm bath and add the entire treatment to the running water.
3. Soak for at least 15 minutes. Use caution when getting out of the bathtub, as it may be slippery.
4. Repeat this treatment once a day as needed.

SOOTHING BACKACHE MASSAGE BLEND

MAKES 10 TREATMENTS

Rosemary, sage, and thyme essential oils are rich in carvacrol and thymol, two natural compounds that aid in muscle relaxation; lavender and Roman chamomile enhance this synergistic blend, and ginger acts as a natural analgesic.

½ ounce carrier oil
6 drops lavender essential oil
4 drops ginger essential oil
4 drops Roman chamomile essential oil
4 drops rosemary essential oil
4 drops sage essential oil
4 drops thyme essential oil

1. In a dark-colored glass bottle, add the carrier oil along with the lavender, ginger, Roman chamomile, rosemary, sage, and thyme essential oils, and shake well to blend.
2. Draw a warm bath and add 4 to 6 drops of the blend to the running water.
3. Soak for at least 15 minutes. Use caution when getting out of the bathtub, as it may be slippery.
4. Towel off, and have a helper apply a small amount of the massage blend to your sore back.
5. Repeat this treatment once a day as needed. Store the bottle in a cool, dark place between uses.

Bad Breath

Halitosis happens to everyone at some point. Bad breath is sometimes caused by the foods you eat, but bacteria is more often the culprit. Brushing and flossing at least twice daily removes food particles, preventing bacterial buildup; natural remedies help eliminate even more bacteria. If your breath has changed suddenly and does not respond to improved oral hygiene and natural remedies, see your doctor, as halitosis can be a symptom of an underlying disease.

Keep your mouth moist to help prevent halitosis. Saliva naturally cleanses and refreshes your mouth. Without it, bacteria build up rapidly, increasing the odds that you'll be plagued by offensive breath. Stay hydrated and your breath will automatically be fresher.

CLOVE RINSE

MAKES 30 TREATMENTS

Clove essential oil is a powerful antibacterial agent that leaves a fresh, pleasant scent behind. Children 12 years old or younger should not use this treatment.

1 pint purified water
30 drops clove essential oil

1. In a dark-colored glass bottle, add the water and clove essential oil, and shake well to blend.
2. Rinse your mouth with 1 tablespoon, swishing the liquid around the teeth and gargling.
3. Repeat this treatment 2 times a day, after brushing and flossing. Try to make each treatment last for at least 30 seconds. Do not swallow the rinse. Shake the treatment before each use.

LAVENDER-PEPPERMINT PURIFYING DROPS

MAKES 30 TREATMENTS

Lavender essential oil eliminates bacteria, while peppermint essential oil leaves a pleasant fragrance behind. Use this treatment to stop bad breath between brushings; keep the bottle with you to enjoy a treatment anytime. Children should not use this treatment.

2 teaspoons vodka
8 drops lavender essential oil
8 drops peppermint essential oil

1. In a dark-colored glass bottle fitted with an orifice reducer, add the vodka along with the lavender and peppermint essential oils, and shake well to blend.
2. Drip 1 to 3 drops on the tongue or under the tongue.
3. Repeat this treatment up to 6 times a day until symptoms subside. Shake the bottle before each use.

Bee Stings

Bee stings bring swelling, pain, and itching with them. If you are suffering from a minor bee sting or even a few stings at once, these remedies will bring rapid relief. Seek medical attention as soon as possible in the event you have been stung by a swarm of bees, or if you are allergic or suspect that you are allergic to bee stings.

LAVENDER-CHAMOMILE COMPRESS

MAKES 1 TREATMENT

Lavender and German chamomile essential oils are natural antihistamines that double as anti-inflammatory agents. Roman chamomile essential oil can be used instead of German chamomile essential oil in this treatment.

1 pint cold water
2 drops lavender essential oil
2 drops German chamomile essential oil
1 drop carrier oil

1. In a medium glass bowl, add the water along with 1 drop of lavender essential oil and 1 drop of German chamomile essential oil.
2. Using your fingertips, apply 1 drop of lavender essential oil directly to the sting, followed by 1 drop of German chamomile essential oil, then the carrier oil.
3. Submerge a towel in the water, wring it out, and apply the compress to the affected area. Leave the compress in place until it warms to body temperature.
4. Repeat this treatment once an hour for up to 4 hours as needed.

BASIL-PEPPERMINT BEE STING RELIEF

MAKES 1 TREATMENT

Basil and peppermint come together in this remedy to relieve the pain and itching that accompany bee stings.

1 drop basil essential oil
1 drop peppermint essential oil
2 drops carrier oil

1. Run cold water over the affected area for 1 minute, then pat dry.
2. Using your fingertips, apply the basil essential oil, followed by the peppermint essential oil, then the carrier oil.
3. Repeat this treatment once an hour for up to 12 hours as needed.

Bleeding Wound

Some minor wounds bleed profusely. Allowing small wounds to bleed for 30 seconds or so before staunching the blood flow and cleaning the wound can help push dirt and bacteria out of the wound. In the event blood is spurting from an artery or a wound is large or very deep, seek medical attention immediately.

STAUNCH BLEEDING WITH HELICHRYSUM

MAKES 1 TREATMENT

Helichrysum essential oil is a strong hemostatic that can be directly applied to wounds to stop bleeding. Use this treatment for small wounds, like shaving accidents and scratches. Use cypress essential oil if helichrysum isn't on hand.

Helichrysum essential oil
Lavender essential oil

1. Using a dropper, drip the helichrysum essential oil directly into the wound, using enough to cover the wound. Do not rub.
2. After the bleeding stops, using a dropper, drip the lavender essential oil over the helichrysum to help prevent infection.
3. Repeat the application of the lavender essential oil 1 or 2 times a day until the wound heals.

GERANIUM-LEMON COMPRESS

MAKES 1 TREATMENT

Geranium and lemon essential oils help soothe pain and halt inflammation, while tea tree essential oil helps prevent infection. This soothing compress is ideal for shallow cuts and scrapes.

1 pint cold water
1 drop geranium essential oil
1 drop lemon essential oil
1 drop tea tree essential oil

1. In a medium glass bowl, add the water along with the geranium, lemon, and tea tree essential oils.
2. Submerge a towel in the water, wring it out, and apply the compress to the affected area. Leave the compress in place until it warms to body temperature.
3. Do not repeat this treatment after a scab has formed.

Blister

Small pockets of fluid usually caused by friction, burning, freezing, infection, or chemical exposure, blisters normally affect the upper layer of the skin, causing pain that can sometimes be severe. Allow blisters to remain intact, if possible, as the skin is a natural barrier to infection. Severe blistering caused by burns, chemical exposure, freezing, and infection may not respond well to natural remedies. Seek medical attention as necessary.

LAVENDER-MYRRH COMPRESS

MAKES 1 TREATMENT

Follow this treatment by applying a donut-shaped blister bandage or some moleskin around the blister, making sure the sticky part of the covering does not touch the blister.

1 pint cold water
3 drops lavender essential oil
3 drops myrrh essential oil
2 drops carrier oil

1. In a medium glass bowl, add the water along with 2 drops of lavender essential oil and 2 drops of myrrh essential oil.
2. Using your fingertips, apply 1 drop of lavender essential oil to the blister, followed by 1 drop of myrrh essential oil, then the carrier oil.
3. Submerge a towel in the water, wring it out, and apply the compress to the affected area. Leave the compress in place until it warms to body temperature.
4. Dry the area before applying a cushioned bandage.
5. Repeat this treatment every 4 hours as needed.

TEA TREE BLISTER SOAK

MAKES 1 TREATMENT

Use this remedy for foot blisters that have broken open or have been drained. Use eucalyptus, lavender, or myrrh essential oil if tea tree essential oil isn't on hand.

4 cups cool water
10 drops tea tree essential oil

1. In a large shallow glass or ceramic basin, add the water and tea tree essential oil, and stir to combine.
2. Soak the foot for 15 minutes, then pat it dry, allowing the blister to air-dry.
3. Repeat this treatment 1 or 2 times a day until the blistered area has healed. To speed the healing process, keep the affected area exposed to open air for as long as possible.

Bloating

Abdominal bloating causes mild to severe discomfort, pressure, and an increase in the abdomen's diameter. In many cases, bloating occurs due to overeating, excessive intake of gas-producing foods, or constipation. Bloating can be a symptom of bowel obstructions, food allergies, and some serious diseases. Seek medical intervention if symptoms worsen or do not improve with both time and the application of natural remedies.

LEMON-ROSEMARY RELIEF

MAKES 1 TREATMENT

Lemon essential oil is a fast-acting natural diuretic, and both peppermint and rosemary essential oils help soothe the discomfort that accompanies bloating.

6 drops carrier oil
2 drops lemon essential oil
2 drops peppermint essential oil
2 drops rosemary essential oil

1. In a small glass bowl, add the carrier oil along with the lemon, peppermint, and rosemary essential oils, and stir to combine.
2. Using your fingertips, apply the blend on the abdomen, and massage it into the skin.
3. Lie on your left side for 15 minutes, relaxing as you breathe in the scent of the essential oils.

Body Odor

Body odor usually occurs when skin bacteria combine with sweat. However, it can occur after the ingestion of pungent foods such as onions and garlic. In most cases, body odor is a benign condition that's more embarrassing and annoying than it is dangerous. In some cases, though, body odor can be indicative of an underlying disease such as cancer, liver or kidney failure, or the spread of infection. If body odor is persistent and fails to respond to improved hygiene and natural treatments, see your doctor for diagnosis.

EUCALYPTUS SALVE

MAKES 10 TREATMENTS

Eucalyptus essential oil fights body odor by thwarting the bacteria that cause it. In addition, it leaves a pleasant fragrance behind. Use this salve on the underarms, feet, and other problem areas.

2 tablespoons carrier oil
30 drops eucalyptus essential oil

1. In a dark-colored glass bottle fitted with an orifice reducer, add the carrier oil and eucalyptus essential oil, and shake well to blend.
2. Using your fingertips or a cotton ball, apply a small amount of the blend to the problem areas.
3. Repeat this treatment up to 3 times a day. Store the bottle in a cool, dark place between uses.

COOLING LAVENDER-MINT POWDER

MAKES 30 TREATMENTS

Lavender essential oil fights the bacteria that contribute to body odor, while both lavender and mint essential oils leave a pleasant, refreshing fragrance behind. Use this powder all over your body, or apply it to problem areas. You may also sprinkle it into your shoes between uses, but be sure to shake it out before the next wearing.

1 cup baking soda
30 drops lavender essential oil
30 drops of peppermint or spearmint essential oil

1. In a medium glass bowl, add the baking soda along with the lavender and mint essential oils, and stir to combine.
2. Pour the mixture into a glass or ceramic sugar shaker, and apply it to problem areas.
3. Repeat this treatment as needed.

Boil

A boil is a deep, localized infection that typically begins as a sore, reddened area approximately a half inch across. Within four to seven days, the lump in the boil's center turns white from pus that has accumulated beneath the skin. Boils often respond well to natural treatment; however, some will worsen despite treatment and require medical intervention. See your doctor if a fever or swollen lymph nodes develop, and seek medical attention if the pain worsens or redness radiates from the boil, if additional boils appear in the area, or if the boil fails to drain.

LAVENDER-TEA TREE SOAK

MAKES 1 TREATMENT

Lavender and tea tree essential oils fight bacteria, while the warmth of a bath draws the boil to a head and promotes faster healing.

11 drops lavender essential oil
11 drops tea tree essential oil

1. Draw a warm bath and add 10 drops of lavender essential oil and 10 drops of tea tree essential oil to the running water.
2. Soak for at least 15 minutes. Use caution when getting out of the bathtub, as it may be slippery.
3. After toweling off, apply the remaining 1 drop of lavender essential oil and 1 drop of tea tree essential oil directly to the boil to speed the healing process, if desired.
4. Repeat this treatment 2 to 4 times a day until the boil ruptures and drains.

LAVENDER-FRANKINCENSE COMPRESS

MAKES 1 TREATMENT

Lavender and frankincense essential oils help stop bacterial activity, and the heat of a compress helps promote drainage.

1 pint hot water
1 drop lavender essential oil
1 drop frankincense essential oil
2 drops carrier oil

1. In a medium glass bowl, add the hot water.
2. Using your fingertips, apply the lavender essential oil to the boil, followed by the frankincense essential oil, then the carrier oil.
3. Submerge a towel in the water, wring it out, and apply the compress to the affected area. Leave the compress in place for at least 10 minutes or until it cools to body temperature.
4. Repeat this treatment up to 6 times a day until the boil has ruptured and drained.

Brittle Hair

Brittle hair is caused by excess exposure to heat, chemicals such as chlorine, or excessive processing such as dyes, straighteners, or perms. Breakage happens often, as do tangling and unmanageability. Prevent brittle hair by sticking to a natural hair care regimen.

GERANIUM-ROSEMARY HAIR MASQUE

MAKES 1 TREATMENT

Geranium and rosemary essential oils help increase circulation and stimulate hair follicles to release more natural oils. Help hair improve faster by avoiding chemicals and hot styling tools.

1 tablespoon jojoba essential oil
6 drops geranium essential oil
6 drops rosemary essential oil

1. In a small glass bowl, combine the jojoba carrier oil along with the geranium and rosemary essential oils, and stir to combine.
2. Using your fingertips, apply the blend to a dry scalp, and massage it gently through the hair.
3. Allow the masque to remain in place for 30 to 60 minutes, then wash the hair as usual.
4. Repeat this treatment 3 times a week until the hair has returned to normal.

SANDALWOOD SPRITZ

MAKES 24 TREATMENTS

Sandalwood essential oil helps promote healthy hair by stimulating the scalp to produce more sebum, which is a natural oil that gives hair its glossy appearance. As a bonus, this spritz smells fantastic.

2 ounces purified water
10 drops argan carrier oil
20 drops sandalwood essential oil

1. In a dark-colored glass bottle fitted with a spray top, add the water, argan carrier oil, and sandalwood essential oil, and shake well to blend.
2. Generously spray wet or dry hair with the blend and allow to dry.
3. Repeat this treatment up to 3 times a day. Shaking the bottle before each use.

Broken Capillaries

Broken or swollen capillaries may occur anywhere on the body but are frequently seen on the nose and cheeks. Capillaries are tiny blood vessels that supply the skin and other organs with oxygen and nutrients while removing waste. When they break or swell, they look like tiny pink, red, or purple threads lying just beneath the skin's surface. If natural remedies do not bring the level of improvement you desire, consider seeing a dermatologist.

HELICHRYSUM SALVE

MAKES 12 TO 24 TREATMENTS

Helichrysum, lavender, and cypress essential oils help constrict blood vessels and reduce the appearance of broken or swollen capillaries. Start this treatment as soon as you notice a problem for best results.

20 drops helichrysum essential oil
16 drops lavender essential oil
12 drops cypress essential oil

1. In a dark-colored glass bottle fitted with an orifice reducer, add the helichrysum, lavender, and cypress essential oils, and shake well to blend.
2. Using your fingertips, apply 2 to 4 drops of the blend to the affected area, rubbing lightly. If applying cosmetics, wait until the essential oils have been absorbed.
3. Repeat this treatment 2 times a day until the broken capillaries fade.

SOOTHING FACIAL COMPRESS

MAKES 1 TREATMENT

Geranium and lemongrass essential oils soothe skin and promote a glowing, healthy look, while cypress, helichrysum, and lavender essential oils help constrict blood vessels.

8 drops argan carrier oil

3 drops helichrysum essential oil

2 drops lavender essential oil

1 drop cypress essential oil

1 drop geranium essential oil

1 drop lemongrass essential oil

1 pint cold water

1. In a small glass bowl, add the argan carrier oil along with the helichrysum, lavender, cypress, geranium, and lemongrass essential oils, and stir to combine.
2. Using your fingertips, apply the entire treatment to your freshly washed face.
3. In a medium glass bowl, add the water.
4. Submerge a towel in the water, wring it out, and apply the compress to the affected area. Leave the compress in place for 15 minutes or until it warms to body temperature.
5. Rinse the face with cool water before applying cosmetics.
6. Repeat this treatment once a day.

Bronchitis

Bronchitis is an inflammatory disease that affects the respiratory system, causing inflamed bronchial tubes, excess mucus production, and coughing. Acute bronchitis is normally caused by a virus and may accompany an upper respiratory tract infection such as a cold or the flu. It can also occur due to aspiration of liquid or food into the lungs, or following exposure to irritants such as heavy smoke. Cases of acute bronchitis typically last two to three weeks. See your doctor if symptoms do not respond to treatment, as bronchitis symptoms can be an indicator of a more serious underlying disease.

DIFFUSE EUCALYPTUS

Eucalyptus essential oil helps open constricted airways and ease coughing. If you do not have a diffuser, the eucalyptus scent can be inhaled directly from the bottle or used in an aromatherapy pendant, or a few drops can be added to bathwater. If eucalyptus essential oil is not available, you may substitute rosemary essential oil, which also eases bronchitis symptoms. Diffuse eucalyptus essential oil in the area where the sufferer is spending the most time.

EUCALYPTUS-LAVENDER RUB

MAKES 12 TREATMENTS

Eucalyptus, lavender, and tea tree essential oils have antibacterial and antiviral properties that help prevent bronchitis from getting worse. They also soothe inflamed airways. Rosemary essential oil can be substituted for eucalyptus essential oil, if desired.

2 ounces carrier oil
20 drops eucalyptus essential oil
20 drops lavender essential oil
20 drops tea tree essential oil

1. In a dark-colored glass bottle, add the carrier oil along with the eucalyptus, lavender, and tea tree essential oils, and shake well to blend.
2. Using your fingertips, apply about 1 teaspoon of the blend over the chest area, and massage it into the skin before relaxing.
3. Repeat this treatment up to 4 times a day until symptoms subside. Store the bottle in a cool, dark place between uses.

Eucalyptus essential oil is powerful medicine. This humble and inexpensive extract is so effective against bacteria and viruses that it, and a derivative called eucalyptol, are used extensively in modern medicine. You'll find it in many OTC remedies, including cough drops, mouthwashes, and antifungal body powders.

Bruise

Bruises are caused when blood vessels rupture or tear following an impact such as a fall or hard bump. Some bruises are minor and fade on their own within a few days; others are accompanied by temporary soreness and swelling. Some bruises spread in the direction of gravity, while others change colors as they heal. If you suffer from severe bruising, pain, and swelling that continue to worsen 30 minutes or longer after an accident, then a fracture or severe sprain may be present. Seek medical attention promptly if you suspect a serious injury is present.

HELICHRYSUM-CYPRESS COMPRESS

MAKES 1 TREATMENT

Helichrysum and cypress essential oils constrict blood vessels to speed bruise healing, particularly when applied at the first signs of bruising. The cold helps prevent bruises from swelling and spreading.

1 drop helichrysum essential oil
1 drop cypress essential oil
2 drops carrier oil
1 pint cold water

1. Using your fingertips, apply the helichrysum essential oil to the bruise, followed by the cypress essential oil, then the carrier oil.
2. In a medium glass bowl, add the water.
3. Submerge a towel in the water, wring it out, and apply the compress to the affected area. Leave the compress in place for 15 minutes or until it warms to body temperature.
4. Repeat this treatment every 6 hours for up to 24 hours.

BRUISE HEALING BLEND

MAKES 12 TO 36 TREATMENTS

After a bruise stops swelling, it's important to promote circulation to the area, which helps speed the healing process. Lavender, lemongrass, and geranium essential oils combined with helichrysum and cypress essential oils aid in promoting faster bruise healing.

10 drops helichrysum essential oil
8 drops lavender essential oil
6 drops cypress essential oil
6 drops geranium essential oil
6 drops lemongrass essential oil

1. In a dark-colored glass bottle fitted with an orifice reducer, add the helichrysum, lavender, cypress, geranium, and lemongrass essential oils, and shake well to blend.
2. Using your fingertips, apply 1 to 3 drops of the blend to the bruised area.
3. Repeat this treatment 2 or 3 times a day until the bruise is healed.

Bug Bites

Insect bites bring itching, mild pain, and redness with them; some are accompanied by swelling at the bite site. Treat insect bites as soon as possible to minimize the irritation, and ensure that you refrain from scratching bite sites, as this can lead to infection while causing the poison that leads to itchiness to spread away from the bite site.

NEAT TEA TREE TREATMENT

Tea tree essential oil stops the itching and burning associated with bug bites. Its antibacterial property helps ensure no subsequent infection occurs. Use this essential oil neat on adults and children above the age of 12. Dilute tea tree essential oil with an equal amount of carrier oil for use on young children or people with sensitive skin. Dab bug bites with a tiny bit of tea tree essential oil. Repeat this treatment every 1 to 2 hours as necessary.

LAVENDER-PEPPERMINT BUG BLEND

MAKES 48 TREATMENTS

Lavender and peppermint essential oils stop the pain and stinging associated with painful insect bites, including ant bites. Use this blend neat on adults and children above the age of 12. For use on young children or people with sensitive skin, dilute the blend with an equal amount of carrier oil.

24 drops lavender essential oil
24 drops peppermint essential oil

1. In a dark-colored glass bottle fitted with an orifice reducer, add the lavender and peppermint essential oils, and shake well to blend.
2. Using your fingertip, apply 1 drop to each bug bite.
3. Repeat this treatment every 1 to 2 hours as necessary until the itching or pain subsides.

Burn

Minor burns can happen to anyone, and are easy to treat with essential oils. Symptoms of first-degree burns include pain and redness at the injury site, while second-degree burns injure deeper layers of skin and may be accompanied by blisters. Third degree-burns injure all skin layers and underlying tissue, and fourth-degree burns involve deeper structures, including ligaments, muscles, tendons, blood vessels, nerves, and bones. If you suspect a third- or fourth-degree burn, seek emergency medical treatment immediately. Use essential oils on first-degree burns only. Do not use essential oils on second-, third-, or fourth-degree burns.

NEAT LAVENDER TREATMENT

Lavender essential oil is sometimes called a first aid kit in a bottle, and its ability to help heal burns and reduce or even prevent scarring is well known. When applied immediately following a minor burn, it removes the heat and sting. Apply enough lavender essential oil to cover the wound. Repeat this treatment every 4 to 6 hours for up to 24 hours.

Lavender essential oil heals burns fast, often without scarring. This important discovery was made in the early 1900s when French chemist René-Maurice Gattefossé burned his hand in his lab. He plunged it into the nearest container of liquid, which just happened to be lavender essential oil. To his amazement, the pain subsided quickly, and no scarring occurred.

PREVENT SCARRING WITH HELICHRYSUM

As burns start to heal, helichrysum essential oil should be applied to promote further healing. This essential oil is unique in its ability to speed tissue regeneration, which is one reason it is often used to reduce or even prevent scarring. Apply 1 to 3 drops of helichrysum essential oil to the burned area 1 to 3 times per day for up to 1 week.

Canker Sore

Canker sores are small ulcers of the mouth. They are usually round, and are typically gray to white in color with red borders. They are often accompanied by tingling, burning, and soreness. Most respond well to natural treatments with essential oils, and often heal within three to seven days. If sores are persistent, large, or numerous, or if they are accompanied by swollen lymph nodes, a fever, or physical sluggishness, be sure to see your doctor, as they could be symptomatic of an underlying disease.

NEAT CLOVE TREATMENT

Clove essential oil stops the pain and itching that accompany canker sores, and it is a strong antiseptic that promotes healing. Using a cotton swab, apply 1 drop of clove essential oil to the canker sore 3 times a day. If you are sensitive to the essential oil, do not apply clove oil neat; instead, dilute it with a small amount, up to half with carrier oil, or add 1 drop to 1 tablespoon or more of water and use it as a mouth rinse.

HEALING LEMON RINSE

MAKES 10 TREATMENTS

Lemon essential oil offers antimicrobial, antiseptic, immune-protective, and bactericidal properties, making it an excellent choice for treating canker sores.

10 ounces purified water
30 drops lemon essential oil

1. In a dark-colored glass bottle, add the water and lemon essential oil, and shake well to blend.
2. Rinse with 1 ounce of the blend, swishing and gargling for at least 30 seconds.
3. Repeat this treatment 3 times a day until the canker sore heals. Shake the bottle before each use.

Lemons are alkaline rather than acidic. For this reason, they are ideal for treating a variety of issues that other sour, truly acidic substances would harm. Although they have a sour taste attributed to citric acid, lemons contain numerous minerals, including potassium, magnesium, calcium, and selenium. The citric acid is metabolized quickly, while the body retains the minerals.

Chapped Lips

Chapped lips often follow exposure to sun, wind, or salt water. Because lips don't have oil glands, it is important to treat chapping right away to prevent it from becoming worse. Treat yourself to frequent lip-moisturizing treatments to keep chapping at bay.

FOUR-OIL BLEND LIP BALM

MAKES 30 TREATMENTS

Aloe vera oil and neroli, Roman chamomile, rose, and rose geranium essential oils come together to soften and heal rough, dry lips. A roller-ball tube can be purchased from most companies that offer essential oil supplies.

½ ounce aloe vera oil
2 drops rose geranium essential oil
1 drop neroli essential oil
1 drop Roman chamomile essential oil
1 drop rose essential oil

1. In a roller-ball glass tube or dark-colored glass bottle, add the aloe vera oil along with the rose geranium, neroli, Roman chamomile, and rose essential oils, and shake well to blend.
2. Use the roller-ball or your fingertips to apply the lip balm to the lips.
3. Repeat this treatment as needed to bring relief. Keep the balm with you when you're actively using it, or store it in a cool, dark place between uses.

FRANKINCENSE-LAVENDER LIP BALM

MAKES 60 TREATMENTS

Both frankincense and lavender essential oils are renowned for their ability to promote the healing of dry, chapped skin. Choose a thick carrier oil such as jojoba or avocado for best results.

½ ounce carrier oil

30 drops frankincense essential oil

30 drops lavender essential oil

1. In a roller-ball glass tube or dark-colored glass bottle, add the carrier oil along with the frankincense and lavender essential oils, and shake well to blend.
2. Use the roller-ball or your fingertips to apply the lip balm to the lips.
3. Repeat this treatment as needed to bring relief. Keep the balm with you when you're actively using it, or store it in a cool, dark place between uses.

Chicken Pox

Chicken pox is a highly contagious viral disease characterized by prominent pox marks and an itchy red rash. Blisters eventually break open and ooze before scabs form. It is vital that the patient be kept as comfortable as possible to prevent scratching, which can lead to infection and cause scars to form.

LAVENDER-TEA TREE SALVE

MAKES 5 TREATMENTS

Lavender essential oil calms skin and relieves itching, and tea tree essential oil helps prevent the chicken pox from becoming infected. Calamine lotion helps the treatment stick to the chicken pox and takes the place of a carrier oil. If you have more than one sick child, consider doubling this recipe.

1 ounce calamine lotion

3 drops lavender essential oil

3 drops tea tree essential oil

1. In a dark-colored glass bottle, add the calamine lotion along with the lavender and tea tree essential oils, and shake well to blend.
2. Dab the salve on the chicken pox as needed, allowing the treatment to dry before putting on clothes.
3. Repeat this treatment as needed throughout the day to bring relief and prevent scratching.

SOOTHING LAVENDER OATMEAL BATH

MAKES 1 TREATMENT

Oatmeal is renowned for its ability to help stop itching caused by chicken pox, hives, and similar conditions. Lavender essential oil helps calm the itch, too, while helping skin heal. To make future baths easier to prepare, cook extra oatmeal in advance.

2 cups cooked oatmeal
4 drops lavender essential oil

1. Place the oatmeal in a cloth bag.
2. Draw a warm bath and add the lavender essential oil to the running water.
3. Add the oatmeal bag to the water.
4. Soak for at least 15 minutes. Use caution when getting out of the bathtub, as it may be slippery.
5. Repeat this treatment as needed to bring relief.

Chilblains

Also known as pernio, chilblains develop after exposure to cold, damp conditions. Chilblains commonly occur as small, itchy, swollen spots on the fingers, toes, ears, and nose.

SOOTHING OIL LAYERING TREATMENT

MAKES 1 TREATMENT

Helichrysum, lavender, and myrrh essential oils help soothe the discomfort that accompanies chilblains while promoting healing and helping prevent infection.

1 drop lavender essential oil
1 drop myrrh essential oil
1 drop helichrysum essential oil
2 drops carrier oil (3 drops if you have sensitive skin)

1. Using your fingertips, apply the lavender essential oil to the affected area, followed by the myrrh essential oil, then the helichrysum essential oil.
2. Top the essential oils with the carrier oil.
3. Repeat this treatment up to 4 times a day until the chilblains are healed.

SOOTHING ROSE GERANIUM BATH OIL

MAKES 5 TREATMENTS

Warm baths promote circulation, while black pepper, lavender, and rose geranium essential oils promote healing and prevent infection.

2½ ounces calendula carrier oil
6 drops black pepper essential oil
6 drops lavender essential oil
6 drops rose geranium essential oil

1. In a dark-colored glass bottle, add the calendula carrier oil along with the black pepper, lavender, and rose geranium essential oils, and shake well to blend.
2. Draw a warm bath and add 1 tablespoon of the blend to the running water.
3. Soak for at least 15 minutes. Use caution when getting out of the bathtub, as it may be slippery.
4. Repeat this treatment once a day until the chilblains are healed. For additional relief, use your fingertips to apply a few drops of this blend directly to the chilblains after emerging from the tub, if desired. Store the bottle in a cool, dark place between uses.

Chronic Fatigue Syndrome

Chronic fatigue syndrome (CFS) causes intense feelings of tiredness that prevent you from accomplishing normal day-to-day activities. Other symptoms include forgetfulness, difficulty concentrating, and memory loss. Pain, lymph node soreness, fever, and persistent headaches accompany some cases. See your doctor if symptoms do not subside with treatment, or if frequent dizziness or severe depression develops.

DIFFUSE BASIL, FRANKINCENSE, AND PEPPERMINT

Basil, frankincense, and peppermint essential oils are well known for their ability to energize the mind and body; they can also help with headaches when diffused. Choose whichever of these essential oils appeals to you, and diffuse it in the area where you spend the most time. You may also obtain relief by wearing an aromatherapy pendant containing one of these essential oils. Alternate between essential oils for additional relief, paying close attention to which one works best for you.

Improve concentration with peppermint essential oil. In the 1990s, researchers working at the University of Cincinnati discovered that the scent of peppermint helped test subjects improve concentration. Whether you are working on an important project or just hoping to make it through the day, peppermint can help.

THYME MASSAGE OIL

MAKES 10 TREATMENTS

Thyme is an excellent antidote to muscle pain; it is also an excellent memory and concentration aid. Because the herb helps combat depression and eliminate feelings of exhaustion, it is an excellent choice for those suffering from CFS. Add up to 10 drops of lavender essential oil to this blend for an even more relaxing massage.

2 ounces carrier oil
20 drops thyme essential oil

1. In a dark-colored glass bottle, add the carrier oil and thyme essential oil, and shake well to blend.
2. Using your fingertips, apply the blend to the affected areas after bathing or showering, and massage it into the skin.
3. Repeat this treatment 1 to 3 times a day as needed. Store the bottle in a cool, dark place between uses.

Cold

Sniffling, sneezing, congestion, and coughing are some of the most common cold symptoms. More often than not, they're preceded by a sore throat. Caused by a virus for which there is no cure, the common cold is often accompanied by fatigue, headache, and a low fever, although not all of these symptoms may be present. Cold symptoms typically respond very well to treatment with essential oils.

CAMPHOR VAPOR TREATMENT

MAKES 1 TREATMENT

Camphor's strong, penetrating aroma helps clear the lungs, ease coughs, and promote relaxation. This vapor treatment helps deliver it straight to the lungs. It may also be diffused in the room where you spend the most time.

3 cups hot water
2 drops camphor essential oil

1. In a shallow bowl or basin, add the hot water and camphor essential oil.
2. Sit comfortably, tenting your head with a towel over the bowl, and breathe deeply for 3 to 4 minutes, emerging for fresh air as needed.
3. Repeat this treatment once a day during your cold.

EUCALYPTUS-PINE COLD LINIMENT

MAKES 5 TREATMENTS

The penetrating aroma and clearing action of eucalyptus and pine essential oils help eliminate chest congestion while clearing sinuses. This liniment can also be used as a bath oil. Take care when getting out of the bathtub, as it may be slippery.

2½ ounces carrier oil
10 drops eucalyptus essential oil
10 drops pine essential oil

1. In a dark-colored glass bottle, add the carrier oil along with the eucalyptus and pine essential oils, and shake well to blend.
2. Using your fingertips, apply 1 tablespoon of the blend to the chest area, and massage it into the skin. Cover the blend with a soft cloth to aid in penetration and keep the treatment in place.
3. Repeat this treatment up to 3 times a day until symptoms subside.

Colic

Babies who suffer from colic often cry for no obvious reason, particularly during the evening. Colicky babies sometimes have swollen bellies, often accompanied by gassiness; most cry for three hours or longer each day on more than three days per week. Colic often lasts for a few months, and may be brought on by sounds, light, and excess stimulation. Babies who are older than four months and who cry for hours at a time could have an underlying health condition that needs to be diagnosed and treated.

GINGER MASSAGE

MAKES 1 TREATMENT

Ginger is one of the best digestive aids there is. This essential oil helps alleviate nausea, cramping, gas, and bloating, and is ideal for soothing colicky babies. Do not use undiluted ginger essential oil on babies. Ensure the baby stays warm and comfortable during the massage; you may also make a warm compress and place it over the stomach or back after the massage. If the tummy massage recommended here is not practical, try using this remedy to massage the baby's feet, then replace her socks or booties.

1 teaspoon carrier oil
5 drops ginger essential oil

1. In the palm of your hand, add the carrier oil and ginger essential oil, and rub the mixture between your hands to warm it.
2. Using circular motions, lightly massage the baby's abdomen and lower back.
3. Repeat this treatment 2 times a day for 2 days.

SOOTHING DILL BATH

Dill essential oil aids in digestion while easing flatulence, constipation, and hiccups; its aroma helps individuals cope with feelings of being overwhelmed, which can help parents and child alike. Diffuse the essential oil in your home and breathe deep while bathing your baby using this simple remedy. Fill the baby's bathtub with warm water and add 4 drops of dill essential oil. Immerse the baby, massaging him while playing relaxing music or speaking gently. Try to make the bath last for at least 5 minutes. Repeat as needed.

Congestion

Nasal congestion, sinus congestion, and chest congestion often occur simultaneously. Stuffiness, nasal discharge, coughing, and headache are often present, and in some cases, excess mucus causes tickling in the back of the throat. Congestion usually responds well to treatment with essential oils. If congestion is accompanied by severe chest pain, a high fever, neck stiffness, color changes around the mouth and nail beds, or if you are coughing up blood, see your doctor, as a serious illness could be present.

DIFFUSE CAMPHOR

Camphor essential oil is a powerful antiseptic and anti-inflammatory that helps alleviate congestion so well it is often found in commercial preparations. Diffuse camphor essential oil in an area where you spend time to help stop the inflammation that accompanies your congestion and to relieve your symptoms.

EUCALYPTUS DIRECT INHALATION

When directly inhaled, eucalyptus essential oil provides rapid congestion relief. Rub a few drops of eucalyptus essential oil on your hands and cup them over your face before inhaling, or inhale the scent directly from the bottle. Diffusing eucalyptus is another excellent option, as is adding 1 or 2 drops in your bath or to a washcloth placed on the floor of your shower.

Constipation

Infrequent bowel movements, straining, hard stools, and lower abdomen discomfort are among the most common symptoms of constipation. While not normally serious, constipation is uncomfortable, embarrassing, and even debilitating in some cases. If increased water and fiber intake combined with natural remedies do not ease your symptoms, see your doctor, as constipation is sometimes a symptom of a more serious illness.

ROSEMARY MOVEMENT MASSAGE

MAKES 10 TREATMENTS

Lemon, peppermint, and rosemary essential oils soothe abdominal discomfort while promoting circulation; the massage helps stimulate the bowel and should provide relief. Hasten the process by drinking 8 ounces of water or herbal tea hourly, and ensure that your diet is conducive to healthy bowel movements.

2½ ounces carrier oil
30 drops rosemary essential oil
20 drops lemon essential oil
10 drops peppermint essential oil

1. In a dark-colored glass bottle, combine the carrier oil along with the rosemary, lemon, and peppermint essential oils, and shake well to blend.
2. Using your fingertips, apply ½ tablespoon to the lower abdomen, and massage it into the skin in a clockwise direction for 5 to 10 minutes.
3. Repeat this treatment up to 3 times a day until the constipation is relieved.

CASSIA MASSAGE

MAKES 1 TREATMENT

Cassia essential oil can help stimulate bowel movements. Because it can cause irritation, make sure that you conduct a patch test prior to using it on sensitive abdominal skin. If cassia essential oil is not on hand, ginger essential oil can be used in its place.

1 teaspoon carrier oil
5 drops cassia essential oil

1. In a small glass bowl, add the carrier oil and cassia essential oil, and stir to combine.
2. Using your fingertips, apply the blend to the lower abdomen, and massage it into the skin in a clockwise direction.
3. Repeat this treatment once an hour until a bowel movement occurs.

Cough

Coughs are sometimes dry and irritating, though they are often accompanied by mucus. Coughing is a method for removing foreign matter or mucus from the upper airway and lungs, and most coughs subside within three to four days. See your doctor if a chronic cough is present, as it may be a symptom of a serious underlying illness.

DIFFUSE LIME

Lime essential oil helps boost the immune system and ease coughs, sinus congestion, and bronchitis. It has an appealing fragrance that refreshes the mind and lifts feelings of minor depression that can accompany an illness. Diffuse lime essential oil in the room where you spend the most time, or directly inhale its scent from the bottle. You may also enjoy using it with an aromatherapy pendant.

LAVENDER-LEMON GARGLE

MAKES 1 TREATMENT

Lavender, lemon, and peppermint alleviate the discomfort that accompanies a cough, clear congestion, and reduce mucus.

1 ounce lukewarm water
2 drops lavender essential oil
2 drops lemon essential oil
2 drops peppermint essential oil

1. In a small drinking glass, add the water along with the lavender, lemon, and peppermint essential oils, and stir to combine.
2. Swish and gargle with small amounts of the treatment until it is all used. Do not swallow the gargle.
3. Repeat this treatment up to 3 times a day during your illness.

Cradle Cap

Sometimes referred to as honeycomb disease or milk crust, cradle cap is a common ailment that affects infants under the age of one. Cradle cap does not harm a baby and is quite common; it is actually a built-up crust of dead skin cells and skin oil on the scalp.

LAVENDER-TEA TREE BALM

MAKES 3 TREATMENTS

Lavender essential oil calms and soothes irritated skin and helps eliminate bacteria. Tea tree essential oil intensifies the antibacterial effect.

1 tablespoon coconut carrier oil
3 drops lavender essential oil
3 drops tea tree essential oil

1. In a small, dark-colored glass bottle, add the coconut carrier oil along with the lavender and tea tree essential oils, and shake well to blend.
2. Using your fingertips, apply 1 teaspoon or less to the scalp, and massage it into the skin, taking care not to get the oil in the baby's eyes.
3. Allow the oils to absorb, then wash the head with warm water.
4. Repeat this treatment once a day until the cradle cap is gone.

GERANIUM SCALP TREATMENT

MAKES 1 TREATMENT

Geranium essential oil is gentler than lavender and tea tree, and it is effective against the bacteria that cause cradle cap, particularly when combined with brushing. Babies typically enjoy the feeling of having their scalps gently rubbed and brushed, and the geranium essential oil has an uplifting effect that will put you in a positive mood, too.

1 teaspoon sesame carrier oil
2 drops geranium or rose geranium essential oil

1. In the palm of your hand, add the sesame carrier oil and geranium essential oil, and rub the mixture between your hands to warm it.
2. Gently apply the blend to the scalp, massaging it into the skin and taking care not to get the oil in the baby's eyes.
3. Use a very soft baby brush to gently rub the affected area.
4. Repeat this treatment up to 3 times a day until the cradle cap is gone.

Croup

Croup often accompanies a cold, and is characterized by a harsh cough that sounds a bit like a barking seal. Because it causes the voice box, bronchial passages, and windpipe to swell, croup makes breathing difficult and the voice raspy. Most cases respond well to natural remedies. If the croup lasts longer than five days, your child needs to be evaluated by a physician.

CROUP RELIEF RUB

MAKES 1 TREATMENT

Frankincense and peppermint essential oils help soothe congestion and ease the discomfort caused by constant coughing. Double the amount of carrier oil in this treatment if you are using it on an infant.

8 drops carrier oil
2 drops frankincense essential oil
2 drops peppermint essential oil

1. In a dark-colored glass bottle, add the carrier oil along with the frankincense and peppermint essential oils, and shake well to blend.
2. Using your fingertips, apply the rub to the child's chest, back, and bottoms of feet or inside ankles, and massage it into the skin.
3. Repeat the treatment every 1 to 3 hours as needed to relieve coughing. To ensure small children do not transfer the oils from their chests to their eyes, dress them in fitted T-shirts.

CALMING PEPPERMINT BATH

MAKES 1 TREATMENT

Peppermint essential oil calms coughs and eases congestions. This bath allows some of the oil to penetrate the skin while the vapors enter the lungs. Draw a warm bath and add 4 to 6 drops of peppermint essential oil to the running water. Allow the child to relax and play in the tub for at least 15 minutes, taking care to keep the water out of the eyes. If bathing a baby with croup, use just 2 or 3 drops of peppermint essential oil.

Cuts and Scrapes

When cuts and scrapes happen, removing any foreign matter and treating the injury with essential oils can help prevent infection and promote healing. If a cut is very deep, or is accompanied by spurting arterial blood, seek emergency treatment.

COOL LAVENDER COMPRESS

MAKES 1 TREATMENT

Lavender essential oil helps take the sting out of cuts and scrapes while eliminating bacteria. The cool compress provides additional relief and stops swelling.

1 pint cold water

6 drops lavender essential oil

1. In a medium glass bowl, add the water and lavender essential oil.
2. Submerge a towel in the water, wring it out, and apply the compress to the wound. Leave the compress in place until it warms to body temperature.
3. Repeat this treatment, using a clean cloth each time, until the bleeding stops.

TEA TREE FIRST AID SPRAY

MAKES 24 TREATMENTS

Tea tree essential oil stops bacterial activity, making this spray ideal for spritzing on small wounds. First rinse the wound with water or, if not near a water source, irrigate the wound well with the spray for effective cleansing.

4 ounces purified water

40 drops tea tree essential oil

1. In a dark-colored glass spray bottle, add the water and tea tree essential oil, and shake well to blend.
2. Spray the blend on the wound.
3. Allow the wound to air-dry after the treatment.
4. Do not repeat this treatment after a scab forms.

Cysts

A cyst is a closed sac-like or capsule-like structure on the skin. It may be filled with fluid, gaseous material, or semi-solid matter, and may be found anywhere on the body. Cysts may be nearly microscopic, although some can become very large. Most are benign and are caused by blockages. Others are caused by serious diseases, including cancer. See your doctor if a cyst worsens rather than responds to treatment.

NEAT FRANKINCENSE TREATMENT

Frankincense essential oil is a strong antiseptic that also helps promote skin healing. It is most effective when applied neat; however, the treatment can be diluted with an equal amount of a carrier oil prior to use. Wash the cyst with soap and water, then pat the skin dry. Apply 1 or 2 drops of frankincense essential oil, allowing it to penetrate the skin. Repeat this treatment up to 3 times a day as the cyst improves and diminishes.

GRAPEFRUIT-THYME SALVE

MAKES 1 TREATMENT

Grapefruit essential oil aids in clearing toxins and reducing skin's oiliness, and thyme is a strong antiseptic that also acts as a circulatory stimulant.

1 drop grapefruit essential oil
1 drop thyme essential oil
2 drops carrier oil (optional)

1. Using your fingertips, apply the grapefruit essential oil to the cyst, followed by the thyme essential oil, then the carrier oil (if using).
2. Repeat this treatment 4 times a day until symptoms subside.

Dandruff

Itchiness and dry, white flakes that land on your shoulders or collar are indicative of dandruff. This condition occurs when the scalp produces excessive skin cells.

CEDARWOOD CONDITIONER

MAKES 10 TREATMENTS

Cedarwood essential oil relieves itching while eliminating dandruff.

5 ounces natural conditioner
20 drops cedarwood essential oil

1. In a dark-colored bottle, add the conditioner and cedarwood essential oil, and shake well to blend.
2. After shampooing and massaging the scalp, use your fingertips to apply 1 tablespoon of the conditioner to the scalp, and massage it into the skin.
3. Leave the conditioner in place for at least 10 minutes, then rinse with cool water.
4. Repeat this treatment once a day until the dandruff is gone. Store the bottle out of the sun in the shower or in a cupboard between uses.

PATCHOULI SPRITZ

MAKES 20 TREATMENTS

Patchouli essential oil soothes itching while eliminating fungus and bacteria.

4 ounces water
40 drops patchouli essential oil

1. In a dark-colored bottle fitted with a sprayer, add the water and patchouli essential oil, and shake well to blend.
2. Spray the blend on wet or dry hair, focusing on the scalp and problem areas.
3. Repeat this treatment at least once a day. Store the bottle in a cool, dark place.

Dental Care

Taking good care of your teeth doesn't just help you look your best; dental care is also important for maintaining overall health. Most dental problems can be prevented by brushing at least twice daily. Using treatments containing essential oils can help prevent problems, as well.

FLOSS WITH CLOVE

Clove essential oil helps stop bacteria from building up in the mouth. While flossing alone is an excellent habit, clove essential oil is a valuable addition to your daily regimen. Apply 1 drop of clove essential oil to your thumb and forefinger, then rub it on your floss before use. Floss at least once a day for clean, healthy teeth and gums. Rinse your mouth with water after and spit; do not swallow. Do not use clove essential oil with children younger than 12 years old.

PEPPERMINT SWISH

Fresh, clean breath doesn't have to come from commercial preparations. Use this simple trick instead of buying mouthwash for naturally delightful breath. Add 1 or 2 drops of peppermint essential oil to 1 tablespoon of water and swish for 30 seconds after brushing and flossing. Repeat this treatment at least 2 times a day.

Depression

Depression often brings feelings of fatigue, difficulty concentrating, and a lack of enjoyment of things you normally find pleasurable. Mild depression keeps you from functioning well and feeling your best, but with treatment, symptoms usually subside. If depression persists despite natural treatments, seek professional help immediately.

DIFFUSE CLARY SAGE

Clary sage essential oil aids in boosting one's mental outlook, relieving stress, and alleviating tension. It has a calming effect on the nerves and emotions, providing balance and encouraging you to enjoy a more positive take on life in general. Diffuse clary sage essential oil in the area where you spend the most time, or use it with an aromatherapy pendant. This remedy may be used daily and is particularly effective when diffused in the morning while getting ready for the day.

DIFFUSE JASMINE

With its lovely, exotic fragrance, jasmine essential oil soothes the nerves while producing feelings of optimism and confidence. It also has a wonderful restorative effect that helps revive tired senses in a gentle, relaxed manner. Diffuse jasmine essential oil in the area where you spend the most time, or use it with an aromatherapy pendant. A few drops can be added to your bath or to a washcloth placed on the floor of your shower, if desired.

Dermatitis

Itchy, flaky skin, red, inflamed areas, and bumpy rashes are all common forms of dermatitis. You may have developed contact dermatitis following exposure to an irritant, or your dermatitis could be brought on by exposure to overly dry, warm air. If dermatitis does not subside with treatment, it could be symptomatic of a serious illness such as skin cancer. See your doctor if natural remedies do not bring improvement.

JUNIPER-GERANIUM BATH OIL

MAKES 10 TREATMENTS

Juniper and geranium essential oils are excellent remedies for rashes, hives, and other types of skin trouble.

5 ounces carrier oil
10 drops juniper essential oil
10 drops geranium essential oil

1. In a dark-colored glass bottle, add the carrier oil along with the juniper and geranium essential oils, and shake well to blend.
2. Draw a hot bath and add 1 tablespoon of the blend to the running water.
3. Soak for at least 15 minutes. Use caution when getting out of the bathtub, as it may be slippery.
4. Repeat this treatment once a day until symptoms subside. Store the bottle in a cool, dark place between uses.

SOOTHING HELICHRYSUM-LAVENDER BALM

MAKES 1 TREATMENT

Both lavender and helichrysum essential oils have marvelous healing effects. They soothe itches, alleviate inflammation, and promote healing and the regeneration of healthy tissue. This simple balm is best when applied directly to skin. Individuals sensitive to these essential oils should dilute the balm with an equal amount of a carrier oil.

1 drop helichrysum essential oil
1 drop lavender essential oil
2 drops carrier oil (optional)

1. Using your fingertips, apply the helichrysum essential oil to the affected area, followed by the lavender essential oil, then the carrier oil (if using).
2. Repeat this treatment 1 or 2 times a day until the symptoms subside.

Diaper Rash

Diaper rash makes babies miserable. Mild cases are simply red and itchy and respond very quickly to treatment and improved hygiene. More complicated cases can be very sore and involve blistering. If you suspect an infection is developing, see your baby's pediatrician.

CALMING MYRRH BALM

MAKES 15 TREATMENTS

Myrrh essential oil contains antifungal and antibacterial constituents and also has a soothing effect on sore skin.

5 tablespoons coconut carrier oil
1 drop myrrh essential oil

1. In a wide-mouth glass jar with a lid, add the coconut carrier oil and myrrh essential oil, and stir to combine.
2. Using your fingertips, apply 1 teaspoon of the balm to the baby's clean, dry bottom after a diaper change.
3. Repeat this treatment after each diaper change until symptoms subside. If desired, this treatment can be continued as a preventive measure.

SOOTHING LAVENDER-CHAMOMILE BABY BALM

MAKES 30 TREATMENTS

Lavender and chamomile essential oils soothe and heal tender skin, while coconut carrier oil creates a barrier against further irritation. Jojoba oil can be substituted as a carrier oil if coconut oil isn't available.

10 tablespoons coconut carrier oil
1 drop lavender essential oil
1 drop Roman chamomile essential oil

1. In a wide-mouth glass jar with a lid, add the coconut carrier oil along with the lavender and Roman chamomile essential oils, and stir to combine.
2. Using your fingertips, apply 1 teaspoon of the balm to the baby's clean, dry bottom after a diaper change.
3. Repeat this treatment after each diaper change until symptoms subside. If desired, this treatment can be continued as a preventive measure.

Diarrhea

Most people have suffered from loose, watery stools, abdominal cramping, and the sense of urgency that accompanies diarrhea. Diarrhea is typically caused by a virus, although dietary indiscretion can also be a contributing factor. Most cases of diarrhea are temporary, lasting no longer than 24 hours and responding well to treatment. If diarrhea persists beyond 24 hours, contains blood, undigested food, or mucus, or is accompanied by vomiting that prevents fluid intake, seek emergency treatment.

MASSAGE WITH FENNEL

MAKES 1 TREATMENT

Fennel essential oil has long been a favorite remedy for a variety of digestive complaints, including diarrhea. Because it is slightly diuretic, you should drink plenty of clear liquids when using it.

1 tablespoon carrier oil
4 drops fennel essential oil

1. In a small glass bowl, add the carrier oil and fennel essential oil, and stir to combine.
2. Using your fingertips, apply the blend to the abdomen, and massage it into the skin.
3. Repeat this treatment up to 3 times a day until symptoms subside.

Dry Skin

Scaling, itchiness, redness, and a rough, ashy appearance accompany dry skin. Often, exposure to harsh environmental conditions causes or complicates dry skin, so be certain to reduce exposure, if possible. These natural moisturizers soothe and heal; increasing fluid intake may bring relief, too.

BALANCING PALMAROSA BLEND

MAKES 1 TREATMENT

Palmarosa essential oil moisturizes and balances the skin while promoting skin cell production. It is great for treating dermatitis, and it is also an excellent weapon in the battle against dry skin that can occur on elbows, knees, hands, and feet.

3 drops palmarosa essential oil
3 drops carrier oil

1. Using your fingertips, apply the palmarosa essential oil to the affected area, followed by the carrier oil.
2. Repeat the treatment 2 or 3 times a day until dry skin is no longer a problem.

LAVENDER-PATCHOULI BATH OIL

MAKES 1 TREATMENT

Both lavender and patchouli soothe inflamed skin and promote healing and overall dermatological health. You can enjoy this oil in a bath or smooth it over large areas of dry, rough skin anytime.

2 tablespoons carrier oil
4 drops lavender essential oil
4 drops patchouli essential oil

1. In a small glass bowl, add the carrier oil along with the lavender and patchouli essential oils, and stir to combine.
2. Draw a warm bath and add the entire treatment to the running water.
3. Soak for at least 15 minutes. Use caution when getting out of the bathtub, as it may be slippery.
4. Repeat this treatment once a day until symptoms subside.

Ear Infection

Ear infections happen when fluid becomes trapped inside the middle ear. Symptoms include ear pain, redness, and earaches. Use these natural remedies to treat minor ear infections, and watch for signs the remedies are not working, including persistent fever and thick, yellowish fluid coming from the ears. If an ear infection is getting worse rather than improving, see a doctor for antibiotics.

TREAT WITH TAGETES

MAKES 1 TREATMENT

Tagetes essential oil is a powerful antimicrobial agent that also brings relief by soothing the pain associated with ear infections.

1 drop tagetes essential oil
1 drop carrier oil

1. Using a clean glass dropper, pick up 1 drop each of tagetes essential oil and the carrier oil.
2. Drip the oil into the affected ear canal.
3. Lay on your opposite side or plug the outside of the ear canal with a cotton ball for 5 minutes after the treatment to prevent the oil from running out.
4. Repeat this treatment 2 or 3 times a day until the ear returns to normal.

EARACHE PAIN RELIEF RUB

MAKES 1 TREATMENT

Clove essential oil penetrates and soothes to provide relief from pain. This treatment is wonderful for using alongside prescription antibiotics, as it offers comfort while you're waiting for the drugs to take effect. If the earache is accompanied by throat pain, combine 2 drops of clove essential oil with 1 tablespoon of water and gargle. Do not swallow the clove essential oil, and do not use the gargle with children younger than 12 years old.

½ teaspoon carrier oil
2 drops clove essential oil

1. In a small glass bowl, add the carrier oil and clove essential oil, and stir to combine.
2. Using your fingertips, apply the blend around the ear and neck, and massage it into the skin.
3. Repeat this treatment every few hours as necessary.

Eczema

Eczema is characterized by patches of red, itchy, inflamed skin. In most cases, itchiness precedes the flaking and rash, which typically appear on the legs, hands, face, and neck. In children, eczema may also affect the inner knees and elbows. Seek medical treatment if the condition does not improve within a week.

CALMING CARROT SEED

Carrot seed essential oil has both calming and antiseptic properties; it is ideal for many problematic skin conditions, including eczema. With regular use, your skin will become softer, smoother, and healthier.

2 drops carrot essential oil

2 drops jojoba carrier oil

1. Using your fingertips, apply the carrot essential oil to the affected area, followed by the jojoba carrier oil.
2. Repeat this treatment 1 or 2 times a day as needed.

SOOTHING COMPRESS

MAKES 1 TREATMENT

Juniper and geranium essential oils soothe itchy, inflamed skin and promote healing, and the cool compress helps intensify their effects.

1 pint cold water

4 drops geranium essential oil

4 drops juniper essential oil

1. In a medium glass bowl, add the water along with the geranium and juniper essential oils.
2. Submerge a towel in the water, wring it out, and apply the compress to the affected area. Leave the compress in place until it warms to body temperature.
3. Repeat this treatment up to 4 times a day, using a fresh cloth each time, until the skin heals.

Edema

Edema, or fluid buildup, often accompanies other illnesses, ranging from tendinitis to diabetes. Some cases accompany minor problems such as insect bites or contact with poison ivy; others come with pregnancy, immobility, or lymphedema. Try these natural remedies with localized occurrences. If they do not bring relief, see your doctor, as edema can be indicative of a serious underlying condition.

FENNEL MASSAGE OIL

MAKES 1 TREATMENT

Fennel helps clear the body of toxins and promotes the release of built-up fluid. Double or triple this recipe to make enough to treat larger areas of edema.

1 teaspoon carrier oil
4 drops fennel essential oil

1. In a small glass bowl, add the carrier oil and fennel essential oil, and stir to combine.
2. Using your fingertips, apply the blend to the affected areas, and massage it into the skin.
3. Repeat this treatment 1 or 2 times a day until symptoms subside.

GERANIUM-GRAPEFRUIT BATH

MAKES 1 TREATMENT

Grapefruit essential oil is a strong diuretic that helps alleviate edema, and geranium essential oil soothes the skin that has been stretched to its limit. You may also use this blend as a massage oil for addressing edema.

2 tablespoons carrier oil
6 drops geranium essential oil
4 drops grapefruit essential oil

1. In a small glass bowl, add the carrier oil along with the geranium and grapefruit essential oils, and stir to combine.
2. Draw a warm bath and add the entire treatment to the running water.
3. Soak for at least 15 minutes. Use caution when getting out of the bathtub, as it may be slippery. Towel off gently.
4. Repeat this treatment once a day until symptoms subside.

Emotional Wellness

Emotional wellness is about more than simply handling life's stresses; it is also about being in tune with your thoughts and feelings, and understanding how they contribute to your behaviors. Essential oils can play a major part in emotional well-being.

FIND BALANCE WITH CASSIA

Cassia essential oil has a sweet, spicy aroma. Credited with imparting both physical and emotional stamina, it reduces irritability and brings on a feeling of contented relaxation, without causing drowsiness. Many people find that cassia is an irritant when applied topically, so stay on the safe side by enjoying its aromatherapeutic effects. Inhale the aroma of cassia essential oil directly or diffuse it in a room you spend the most time in. This essential oil can also be effective in an aromatherapy pendant.

LOWER STRESS WITH PATCHOULI

Patchouli essential oil interacts with the limbic system to impart an almost immediate calming effect. Use it any way you like; it is beneficial to skin health and may be enjoyed topically. Inhale the aroma of patchouli essential oil directly when feeling stressed, or diffuse it in your home or workspace. Placed inside an aromatherapy pendant, it offers a constant, uplifting presence.

Erectile Dysfunction

Often referred to as impotence, erectile dysfunction is the inability to achieve or maintain an erection. Some causes include chronic illness, medications, poor blood flow, fatigue, or excess alcohol intake.

JASMINE MASSAGE OIL

MAKES 20 TREATMENTS

Jasmine essential oil has an excellent reputation as a natural aphrodisiac. It also helps ease the nervousness and anxiety that often accompany erectile dysfunction, replacing those feelings with a sense of confidence and euphoric bliss.

4 ounces carrier oil
40 drops jasmine essential oil

1. In a dark-colored glass bottle, add the carrier oil and jasmine essential oil, and shake well to blend.
2. Using your fingertips, apply about ½ tablespoon to the chest, shoulders, arms, legs, and back, and massage it into the skin. Share the oil with a partner if you like.
3. Repeat this treatment once a day. Store the bottle in a cool, dark place between uses.

PATCHOULI MASSAGE OIL

MAKES 20 TREATMENTS

Not only is patchouli essential oil an excellent tonic for the skin, it also has a balancing effect on the mind, promoting a relaxed state of happiness while creating a romantic atmosphere. Use it in conjunction with conventional treatment to enhance amorous encounters.

4 ounces carrier oil
40 drops patchouli essential oil

1. In a dark-colored glass bottle, add the carrier oil and patchouli essential oil, and shake well to blend.
2. Using your fingertips, apply about ½ tablespoon to the chest, shoulders, arms, legs, and back, and massage it into the skin. Share the oil with a partner if you like.
3. Repeat this treatment once a day. Store the massage oil in a cool, dark place between uses.

Fainting

Fainting is a brief, sudden loss of posture and consciousness caused by reduced blood flow to the brain. Pregnancy, anemia, age, and dehydration are some contributors; others include heart conditions and diabetes. Fainting may also happen due to stress, hunger, fear, anxiety, or pain; if it happens without provocation, an underlying condition may be present. See your doctor to rule out a serious illness if fainting occurs more than once.

INHALE PEPPERMINT

Peppermint essential oil promotes mental alertness and can help a fainting victim quickly. Loosen any tight clothing, raise the victim's feet above head height, and place the open bottle of peppermint essential oil under the nose, taking care not to allow the essential oil to come into contact with the skin. Allow the victim to take several breaths before removing the bottle. Use lavender or rosemary essential oil if you don't have peppermint on hand.

Fibromyalgia

Often misdiagnosed and misunderstood, fibromyalgia is a common musculoskeletal disorder characterized by widespread joint and muscle pain, fatigue, depression, and an inability to concentrate. Essential oils can help provide physical and emotional relief for the discomfort that accompanies fibromyalgia.

RENEW WITH JASMINE

Because fibromyalgia takes an emotional toll, it's important to do all you can to keep stress and depression at bay. Jasmine essential oil is one of the best choices for alleviating emotional upset naturally. To enjoy the aromatherapeutic effects of jasmine essential oil add 3 to 5 drops to a diffuser, directly inhale its scent from the bottle, or add 1 drop to an aromatherapy pendant. You can also add 8 to 10 drops to a warm bath. The more methods you choose to employ, the more jasmine essential oil will benefit you.

JASMINE MASSAGE OIL

MAKES 1 OR 2 TREATMENTS

Receive the stress-reducing benefits of jasmine essential oil along with the soothing effects of a gentle massage.

1 ounce carrier oil
3 to 5 drops jasmine essential oil

1. In a dark-colored glass bottle, add the carrier oil and jasmine essential oil, and shake well to blend.
2. Using your fingertips, apply 1 to 2 tablespoons of the blend to the affected area, and massage it gently into the skin.
3. Repeat this treatment once a day as needed.

VETIVER MASSAGE OIL

MAKES 20 TREATMENTS

Vetiver essential oil is a marvelous antidote to general aches and pains, including muscle aches, joint pain, and generalized discomfort. It promotes healthful rest while encouraging a relaxed, positive outlook on life.

4 ounces carrier oil
40 drops vetiver essential oil

1. In a dark-colored glass bottle, add the carrier oil and vetiver essential oil, and shake to blend.
2. Using your fingertips, apply about ½ tablespoon to the affected area, and massage it into the skin.
3. Repeat this treatment once a day as needed. Store the bottle in a cool, dark place between uses.

Flatulence

Gas is produced as the stomach and intestines break food into smaller particles for energy. All people pass gas; however, some foods, beverages, dietary supplements, and medications increase gas production or cause extremely unpleasant odors. Uncomfortable gas that doesn't go away with treatment could indicate the presence of an underlying illness. See your doctor if severe gas persists.

PEPPERMINT MASSAGE OIL

MAKES 1 TREATMENT

Peppermint is an excellent antidote to intestinal gas, bloating, cramping, and flatulence, and its pleasant fragrance may help take your mind off the discomfort.

1 teaspoon carrier oil
5 drops peppermint essential oil

1. In a small glass bowl, add the carrier oil and peppermint essential oil, and stir to combine.
2. Using your fingertips, apply the blend to the abdomen, and massage it into the skin. You may also use this treatment on the soles of your feet, the inner portions of your elbows, and the insides of your ankles.
3. Repeat this treatment once a day as needed.

Fleas

Fleas may come indoors with pets, or they may hitch a ride on socks, shoes, and trouser legs. Treating your home and pets with natural essential oils is a good alternative to chemical solutions.

CITRONELLA CARPET POWDER

MAKES 1 TREATMENT

Fleas love to hide in carpet. Repel them while making cleanup easier with this natural, fresh-smelling carpet powder. Both citronella and lemongrass repel fleas, and borax acts as a chemical-free pesticide.

1 cup borax
20 drops citronella essential oil
10 drops lemongrass essential oil

1. In a medium glass bowl, add the borax along with the citronella and lemongrass essential oils, and stir to combine.
2. Transfer the mixture to a sugar shaker.
3. Sprinkle the powder generously on the carpet.
4. Allow the treatment to remain in place for 1 hour, then vacuum the carpet.
5. Repeat the treatment once a day as needed.

FLEA-FREE PET

Lavender essential oil is a natural flea repellent that can be used instead of toxic topical treatments sold in stores. As an added benefit, lavender kills the fungus and bacteria that cause some pets to emit an unpleasant odor. Apply lavender essential oil directly to your dog or cat by sprinkling 1 to 3 drops onto your hands and rubbing it in the fur. Repeat this treatment daily during flea season.

Flu

The flu is a viral infection that affects the lungs, throat, and sinuses. Its symptoms are much like those of the common cold, but they are often preceded by aches, chills, and fever. The flu hits faster and harder than a cold does. It typically begins with a run-down feeling whereas a cold normally starts with a sore throat or runny nose. Fortunately, many of the same essential oils that work well for colds are equally effective against the flu. In both cases, the faster you take action, the less severe your symptoms are likely to be and the sooner you'll feel better.

IMMUNE-BOOSTING BATH

MAKES 1 TREATMENT

Tea tree, lavender, and lemon essential oils help boost immunity and act as antiviral agents that help keep the virus from growing out of control.

1 tablespoon carrier oil
6 drops tea tree essential oil
5 drops lavender essential oil
2 drops lemon essential oil

1. In a small glass bowl, add the carrier oil along with the tea tree, lavender, and lemon essential oils, and stir to combine.
2. Draw a hot bath and add the entire treatment to the running water.
3. Soak for at least 15 minutes. Use caution when getting out of the bathtub, as it may be slippery.
4. Repeat this treatment once a day until the symptoms subside.

DIFFUSE EUCALYPTUS

Eucalyptus essential oil can help stop the spread of the flu virus when diffused. It also helps reduce inflammation and discomfort in flu sufferers. Add 2 or 3 drops of eucalyptus essential oil to a diffuser and place it in the room where you spend the most time. If you do not have a diffuser, blend 20 drops of eucalyptus essential oil with ½ cup of water in a water bottle and spritz the mixture into the air. Repeat the spray every 30 minutes or so to help keep the air saturated with particles of essential oil.

Folliculitis

Folliculitis is a painful condition characterized by infected hair follicles. Commonly affecting the scalp, face, groin, and thighs, it is typically caused by bacteria, fungus, or yeast, and is complicated by tight clothing and shaving. Folliculitis typically responds well to treatment with essential oils and the removal of irritants; however, you should seek medical attention if the problem worsens or fails to respond.

NEAT LAVENDER TREATMENT

Lavender essential oil is a strong antibacterial agent that pulls double duty by soothing inflamed skin and reducing swelling. Apply lavender essential oil neat to areas with folliculitis, using just enough to cover the affected area, and allow the skin to absorb the essential oil before putting on clothes. Repeat this treatment 2 times a day until the problem has been resolved.

NEAT YLANG-YLANG TREATMENT

Ylang-ylang essential oil is a strong antiseborrheic and antiseptic that soothes and balances skin and helps eliminate bacterial infections. Apply ylang-ylang essential oil neat to areas with folliculitis, using just enough to cover the affected area, and allow the skin to absorb the essential oil before putting on clothes. Repeat this treatment 2 times a day until the problem has been resolved.

Foot Odor

Foot odor occurs when bacteria or fungi invade socks, shoes, and foot skin. Most foot odor disappears with treatment and improved hygiene. Medical intervention is not normally necessary. Be sure to keep your feet dry, and remove your shoes and socks when possible to help prevent bacterial buildup. Do not use this treatment with children.

PEPPERMINT FOOT SPRAY

MAKES 24 TREATMENTS

Peppermint essential oil cools and soothes hot, tired feet while leaving a pleasant fragrance behind. Use this delightful foot spray anytime your feet feel less than fresh.

½ cup vodka
20 drops peppermint essential oil

1. In a spray bottle, add the vodka and peppermint essential oil, and shake well to blend.
2. Spray the feet after showering to help prevent bacterial buildup.
3. Repeat this treatment at least once a day until the foot odor disappears.

TEA TREE FOOT POWDER

MAKES 24 TREATMENTS

Tea tree essential oil is a powerful antifungal agent that helps keep odor-causing germs from growing out of control. Baking soda helps absorb any odors that do develop.

1 cup baking soda
20 drops tea tree essential oil

1. In a sugar shaker, add the baking soda and tea tree essential oil, and stir to combine.
2. Shake the powder onto dry feet just before putting on shoes and socks. Alternately, pour about 1 teaspoon of powder into each of your socks before slipping them on your feet, and treat shoes with the powder between uses.
3. Repeat this treatment once a day until the foot odor disappears.

Gastroesophageal Reflux (GERD)

Gastroesophageal reflux (GERD) is characterized by persistent heartburn, a sore throat, nausea, food regurgitation, chest pain, and a chronic cough. GERD often responds well to natural remedies paired with the removal of triggers such as fatty or spicy foods. If symptoms persist or worsen, see your doctor, as it can lead to more serious gastrointestinal conditions.

DIGEST WITH FRANKINCENSE

Frankincense essential oil is a well-respected digestive agent that helps soothe and calm the body and mind. Massage a few drops of frankincense essential oil onto your throat and upper chest area when experiencing a GERD incident. Sit up straight or lie on your left side to help keep the gastric acid contained while the frankincense essential oil goes to work.

Gingivitis

Gingivitis is a common form of periodontal disease characterized by swelling and inflammation of the gum tissue that surrounds the teeth. The disease is often accompanied by halitosis, tenderness, and bleeding. Without improved oral hygiene, gingivitis often progresses, contributing to tooth decay and subsequent tooth loss.

SOOTHE INFLAMMATION WITH CLOVE

Clove essential oil stops dental pain, reduces inflammation, and kills bacteria associated with gingivitis. Using a cotton swab, dab clove essential oil directly onto inflamed gum tissue. Wait 15 minutes before eating or drinking anything, and rinse with water and spit first. Do not swallow clove essential oil. Repeat the treatment at least once a day until the inflammation has cleared up. Dilute the essential oil with an equal amount of a carrier oil for use with children younger than 12 years old.

SWISH WITH MYRRH

MAKES 1 TREATMENT

Myrrh essential oil kills bacteria and soothes inflammation. While not as potent as clove essential oil, it can play an important role in good dental hygiene.

1 tablespoon purified water
3 drops myrrh essential oil

1. In a small drinking glass, add the water and myrrh essential oil, and stir to combine.
2. Swish thoroughly with the blend. Try to make the treatment last for at least 30 seconds before spitting. Do not eat or drink anything for at least 15 minutes.
3. Repeat this treatment 2 or 3 times a day even after gingivitis has been eliminated to help prevent recurrence of the disease.

Grief

Grief is a normal but painful process most people go through when a loved one dies or a relationship ends. Many people also experience deep grief following the loss of a companion animal. Essential oils can facilitate the grieving process by bringing comfort and relief.

DIFFUSE WITH BENZOIN

Benzoin essential oil calms the nervous system, comforting the bereaved and easing the emotional exhaustion that often accompanies the loss of a loved one. Its fragrance is slightly reminiscent of vanilla—sweet, warm, and welcoming. Diffuse benzoin essential oil in areas where people gather or where you spend the most time. You may also inhale its scent directly or place it in an aromatherapy pendant.

RELAX WITH A ROSE BATH

MAKES 1 TREATMENT

Rose essential oil soothes depression, grief, nervous tension, stress, anger, and fear— all emotions that are commonly felt during the grieving process. Help yourself through this difficult time by using rose essential oil in a variety of ways: diffuse it, use it like perfume, and relax with it while bathing.

1 tablespoon carrier oil
10 drops rose essential oil

1. In a small glass bowl, add the carrier oil and the rose essential oil, and stir to combine.
2. Draw a warm bath and add the entire treatment to the running water.
3. Soak for at least 15 minutes. Use caution when getting out of the bathtub, as it may be slippery.
4. Repeat this treatment once a day as needed.

Gum Disease

Gum disease is often preceded by gingivitis, and can have a number of symptoms, including swelling, bright red or purple color, pain, bleeding, bad breath, and a receding gum line. Some contributors are tobacco use, failure to brush and floss, and poor diet. If gum disease does not respond to improved hygiene and treatment, see your dentist.

OIL PULL WITH CLOVE

MAKES 1 TREATMENT

Oil pulling helps remove bacteria, and adding clove essential oil to the carrier oil can help reverse gum disease. To avoid accidental ingestion, do not use this remedy with children younger than 12 years old.

1 tablespoon coconut, olive, or sunflower carrier oil
1 drop clove essential oil

1. In a small drinking glass, add the coconut carrier oil and clove essential oil, and stir to combine.
2. Swish the blend around your cheeks and gums, then use suction to draw the oil through the spaces between your teeth. Keep going for as long as you can; ideally, this treatment will last for at least ten to 15 minutes.
3. Repeat this treatment once a day even after gum disease has been eliminated to help prevent recurrence of the disease.

NEAT MYRRH TREATMENT

Treating with clove essential oil each day is one of the best ways to stop gum disease, but myrrh has powerful antibacterial properties that can help, too. As part of a total dental regimen, use a cotton swab to apply myrrh essential oil to your gums at least once a day until the gums have healed.

Hair Loss

Hair loss often accompanies stress, hormonal changes, illness, and childbirth; certain drugs and cosmetic procedures may contribute to the problem, as well. In some cases, such as in male pattern baldness, hair loss is genetic and inevitable; in other cases, natural remedies may help hair follicles resume normal hair production.

BAY SPRITZ

MAKES 24 TREATMENTS

Bay essential oil has long been used in hair tonics, mostly for its sweet, spicy scent. Because it is a strong antiseptic with astringent properties, it is useful for counteracting hair loss.

4 ounces water
24 drops bay essential oil

1. In a dark-colored glass bottle fitted with a spray top, add the water and bay essential oil, and shake well to blend.
2. Spray the blend onto wet or dry hair to stimulate hair growth, focusing on the scalp.
3. Repeat this treatment 2 times a day. Shake the bottle before each use.

MELISSA HOT OIL TREATMENT

MAKES 1 TREATMENT

Melissa essential oil calms stress and eliminates bacteria. It can play a part in a natural hair restoration program so long as the cause is neither hormonal nor genetic.

2 tablespoons carrier oil
6 drops melissa essential oil

1. In a glass jar, add the carrier oil and the melissa essential oil, and shake well to blend.
2. Place the jar inside a larger jar already filled with steaming hot water. After 5 minutes, remove the small jar and test to make sure the mixture is warm and not too hot.
3. Pour the mixture onto your hair, and massage it into your scalp.
4. Repeat this treatment once every 3 days until hair growth returns.

Hay Fever

Allergic rhinitis, or hay fever, brings watering eyes, a runny nose, and uncontrollable sneezing. Normally caused by tree, grass, or weed pollen, it typically occurs while plants are actively growing. Essential oils effectively soothe hay fever symptoms in most cases; if symptoms persist, you may need to see your doctor for something stronger.

INHALE NIAOULI

Niaouli essential oil is an extremely powerful decongestant with strong antiseptic properties. It is an excellent remedy for alleviating the sudden stuffiness, sneezing, and wheezing that often accompanies a hay fever attack. Place 3 or 4 drops of niaouli essential oil onto a handkerchief or tissue and inhale it when a hay fever attack occurs.

TREAT AIR FILTERS

Air filters act as a first line of defense against the allergens that cause hay fever. Treat them with essential oils to make them even more effective. Drip 5 drops of eucalyptus, lemon balm, or tea tree essential oil on the air filter. The vapors from the essential oils will help you cope better, even if you cannot detect them. At the same time, consider diffusing one or more of these essential oils in your home or workspace.

Headache

Headaches happen to almost everyone from time to time. Often brought on by stress or symptomatic of another condition such as a cold or the flu, headaches may respond well to treatment with essential oils. If you are suffering from chronic, unexplained headaches, see your doctor, as an underlying condition could be the cause.

DIFFUSE CALAMUS

Calamus essential oil acts directly on the nervous system to help ease headaches and promote a refreshed, renewed feeling. Diffuse calamus essential oil at the first sign of a headache or use it in an aromatherapy pendant. A few drops can also be placed on a cotton ball and held or placed close enough to allow the vapors to go to work.

INCREASE CIRCULATION WITH A LEMON BATH

MAKES 1 TREATMENT

Lemon essential oil helps improve circulation, which in turn can help ease headaches. Its usefulness as an antirheumatic aids in reducing the stiffness and tension that often contributes to head pain.

1 tablespoon carrier oil
4 drops lemon essential oil

1. In a small glass bowl, add the carrier oil and the lemon essential oil, and stir to combine.
2. Draw a hot bath and add the entire treatment to the running water.
3. Soak for at least 15 minutes. Use caution when getting out of the bathtub, as it may be slippery.
4. Repeat this treatment as often as you like.

Healthy Heart Function

Keep your heart healthy, and you are more likely to enjoy a physically comfortable life, greater longevity, and all the good things that accompany a long life well lived.

DIFFUSE YLANG-YLANG

Ylang-ylang essential oil is a hypotensive, meaning it helps promote a decrease in blood pressure. It soothes and relaxes body and mind, easing anxiety and tension while promoting relaxation. Add 3 to 5 drops to a diffuser to achieve the best aromatherapy benefits of ylang-ylang essential oil. Keep cool and calm all day by using it in an aroma-therapy pendant.

SOOTHING PETITGRAIN BATH OIL

MAKES 1 TREATMENT

Petitgrain essential oil is an antispasmodic that helps reduce rapid heartbeat and ease breathing. Inhale it when you are feeling stressed or enjoy even more benefits by relaxing with this wonderfully scented bath. Note that very hot water can cause blood pressure to increase, so it is contraindicated for reducing heart rate.

1 tablespoon carrier oil
4 drops petitgrain essential oil

1. In a small glass bowl, add the carrier oil and the petitgrain essential oil, and stir to combine.
2. Draw a warm bath and add the entire treatment to the running water.
3. Soak for at least 15 minutes. Use caution when getting out of the bathtub, as it may be slippery.
4. Repeat this treatment once a day as needed.

YLANG-YLANG BATH OIL

MAKES 1 TREATMENT

Though not as effective as in a diffuser, ylang-ylang can also be used in baths to relax the mind and body as well as decrease blood pressure.

3 or 4 drops ylang-ylang essential oil

1. Draw a warm bath and add the ylang-ylang essential oil to the running water.
2. Soak for at least 15 minutes. Use caution when getting out of the bathtub, as it may be slippery.
3. Repeat this treatment once a day as needed.

RELAXING YLANG-YLANG MASSAGE OIL

MAKES 2 TO 6 TREATMENTS

Ease anxiety and tension while soothing muscles and reducing blood pressure with ylang-ylang essential oil.

1 ounce carrier oil
10 to 20 drops ylang-ylang essential oil

1. In a small glass bowl, add the carrier oil and ylang-ylang essential oil, and stir to combine.
2. Using your fingertips, apply between 1 teaspoon and 1 tablespoon of the blend to the body, and massage it into the skin.
3. Repeat this treatment once a day as needed.

Healthy Liver Function

The liver is a hard-working organ tasked with toxin removal. Make essential oils part of your plan for maintaining healthy liver function for life.

DETOXIFYING CARROT SEED MASSAGE OIL

MAKES 1 TREATMENT

Carrot seed essential oil is a powerful detoxification agent capable of boosting liver health; as an added benefit, it is an excellent skin balancer. Use this treatment if you've overdone it with rich food or too much alcohol.

1 tablespoon carrier oil
6 drops carrot seed essential oil

1. In a small glass bowl, add the carrier oil and carrot seed essential oil, and stir well to combine.
2. Using your fingertips, apply the blend to the abdomen and middle portion of the back, and massage it into the skin.
3. Repeat this treatment 3 times a day until symptoms subside. Drink a lot of clear liquid all day to flush your system.

DETOXIFYING FENNEL BATH

MAKES 1 TREATMENT

Fennel essential oil is a less powerful detoxifier than carrot seed but is effective nevertheless in combating excess, as it is a strong diuretic and liver tonic. If you've had too much rich food or alcohol, or if you are detoxifying your body for another purpose, you'll find that this remedy helps.

1 tablespoon carrier oil

5 drops fennel essential oil

1. In a small glass bowl, add the carrier oil and fennel essential oil, and stir to combine.
2. Draw a hot bath and add the entire treatment to the running water.
3. Soak for at least 15 minutes. Use caution when getting out of the bathtub, as it may be slippery.
4. Repeat this treatment 3 times a day until symptoms subside. Drink a lot of clear liquid all day to flush your system.

Heartburn

Heartburn starts with a burning sensation in the chest, usually right after eating. It may last for just a few minutes or continue for several hours. In some cases, you may feel as if food is stuck in the middle of your throat or chest, or you may feel burning in your throat. Although heartburn does sometimes cause chest pain, seek medical help immediately if unexplained chest pain is present, as this is one of the chief symptoms of a heart attack.

Stop heartburn by eliminating triggers. Essential oils and other heartburn remedies ease symptoms, but they don't eliminate the cause of heartburn. Notice what sets heartburn symptoms in motion, then eliminate potential triggers until you have discovered the cause. Potential causes include acidic foods, caffeine, and wearing tight clothing that puts pressure on your stomach.

EUCALYPTUS-FENNEL RUB

MAKES 1 TREATMENT

Eucalyptus, fennel, and peppermint essential oils are strong digestive agents that help alleviate nausea and quell other heartburn symptoms. Some people find that peppermint causes heartburn to get worse; if you are one of them, omit it from the treatment.

1 teaspoon carrier oil
2 drops eucalyptus essential oil
2 drops fennel essential oil
1 drop peppermint essential oil

1. In a small glass bowl, add the carrier oil along with the eucalyptus, fennel, and peppermint essential oils, and stir to combine.
2. Using your fingertips, apply the blend to the upper abdominal area, and massage it into the skin.
3. Repeat this treatment up to 3 times a day for up to 1 week.

Heat Rash

Also referred to as prickly heat, heat rash typically affects areas of the body that are covered by clothing. Heat rash looks like tiny pimples, and though it typically affects babies, it can also affect children and adults, particularly in hot, humid climates. Watch for swelling, pus, red streaks, and swollen lymph nodes, along with a fever of 100 degrees Fahrenheit or higher; if any of these occur, infection could be present and medical attention is required.

SKIN-SOOTHING EUCALYPTUS-LAVENDER BATH

MAKES 1 TREATMENT

Eucalyptus, lavender, and baking soda come together in this soothing bath treatment, calming the fierce itch and inflammation that accompany heat rash.

1 cup baking soda
4 drops eucalyptus essential oil
4 drops lavender essential oil

1. In a medium glass bowl, add the baking soda along with the eucalyptus and lavender essential oils, and stir to combine.
2. Draw a warm bath and add the entire treatment to the running water.
3. Soak for at least 15 minutes. Use caution when getting out of the bathtub, as it may be slippery.
4. Repeat this treatment once a day as needed.

COOLING CHAMOMILE-PEPPERMINT MIST

MAKES 24 TREATMENTS

Chamomile and peppermint essential oils calm the itching and inflammation of heat rash; store this mist in the refrigerator between applications for even more cooling power.

4 ounces water
8 drops German chamomile or Roman chamomile essential oil
2 drops peppermint essential oil

1. In a dark-colored glass bottle fitted with a spray top, add the water along with the German chamomile and peppermint essential oils, and shake well to blend.
2. Spray the blend onto the affected area.
3. Repeat this treatment every 2 to 3 hours as needed.

Hemorrhoids

Hemorrhoids are swollen, inflamed veins inside the anal canal that can cause itching and burning, and in some cases, lead to bleeding and pain. Minor hemorrhoids tend to respond well to treatments with essential oil, while severe cases sometimes require surgical intervention. See your doctor if hemorrhoids do not respond to natural remedies.

NEAT GERANIUM TREATMENT

Hemorrhoids are itchy, painful, and swollen. Geranium essential oil addresses all three of these problems by cooling, soothing, and reducing inflammation. Using a cotton pad soaked with 5 or 6 drops of geranium or rose geranium essential oil, swab the affected area 2 or 3 times a day as needed.

FRANKINCENSE-HELICHRYSUM WIPES

MAKES 20 TREATMENTS

Frankincense, helichrysum, and lavender essential oils address itching, burning, inflammation, and pain while promoting healing and reducing swelling. Witch hazel is a strong astringent and aids in shrinking the hemorrhoids while bringing cooling relief.

1 ounce witch hazel
20 drops frankincense essential oil
20 drops helichrysum essential oil
20 drops lavender essential oil

1. In a small glass bowl, add the witch hazel along with the frankincense, helichrysum, and lavender essential oils, and stir to combine.
2. Inside a wide-mouth pint jar, stack 20 cotton pads. Pour the liquid blend over the cotton pads. Cap the jar tightly with a lid and store it in a cool, dark place.
3. Use 1 pad as the final wipe after each bowel movement or any time relief is needed.

Hiccups

Just about everyone gets hiccups, which happen when involuntary spasms cause the diaphragm to contract repeatedly. Hiccups respond well to essential oils, usually subsiding within a few minutes. In some cases, hiccups last for hours; if they continue for 48 hours or longer, seek medical attention, as persistent or intractable hiccups often signal the presence of a serious underlying condition.

DILL HICCUP SALVE

MAKES 1 TREATMENT

Dill essential oil is an effective antispasmodic that helps put a stop to annoying hiccups fast. Drinking warm water helps the treatment work more rapidly.

4 drops carrier oil
2 drops dill essential oil

1. In a small glass bowl, add the carrier oil and dill essential oil, and stir to combine.
2. Using your fingertips, trace a line of the blend along your jaw from one earlobe to the other.
3. Drink a glass of warm water, focusing on the feeling of the water as it makes its way down your throat.
4. Repeat this treatment once if hiccups persist for 5 minutes after first treatment.

CHAMOMILE-SPEARMINT INHALATION

MAKES 1 TREATMENT

Chamomile and spearmint essential oils are effective antispasmodics, and breathing in a paper bag is a common home remedy for hiccups, as it stimulates deep, regular breathing that can calm the diaphragm.

2 drops German chamomile or Roman chamomile essential oil
2 drops spearmint essential oil

1. Dot the German chamomile and spearmint essential oils into the paper bag.
2. Hold the bag over your nose and mouth while slowly inhaling and exhaling through your nose.
3. Continue this treatment until hiccups subside.

Hives

Hives are swollen bumps on the skin and appear suddenly. While hives usually itch, they sometimes sting or burn. The raised patches vary in size, with some being about the diameter of a pencil eraser and others being as large as dinner plates. They can also join at their edges to form much larger areas called plaques. Hives typically respond well to essential oils, but you should seek emergency treatment if they are accompanied by vomiting or shortness of breath, or if home remedies fail to bring relief.

NEAT BASIL TREATMENT

Basil essential oil is an effective analgesic that stops the pain and itching associated with hives, lowering the risk of scratching and causing the problem to worsen. Using a cotton ball, apply a small amount of basil essential oil to each affected area, allowing it to penetrate. Repeat this treatment every 3 to 4 hours as needed.

NEAT MYRRH TREATMENT

Myrrh essential oil has anti-inflammatory and astringent properties that make it ideal for soothing serious itching and addressing the swelling that accompanies hives. Using a cotton ball or your fingertips, apply a small amount of myrrh essential oil to each affected area, allowing it to penetrate. Repeat this treatment every 3 to 4 hours as needed.

Immune Support

A strong immune system is invaluable, standing ready to take action in the event illness strikes. A healthy diet, exercise, quality sleep, good hygiene, and stress management help ensure that your immune system is up to the task of fighting disease whenever the need arises.

ANTIBACTERIAL AND ANTIVIRAL DIFFUSION BLEND

Lavender, tea tree, and thyme essential oils are renowned for their ability to keep sickness at bay. At the very least, this diffusion is likely to lessen symptoms and shorten duration. In a dark-colored glass bottle large enough to hold the amount of the diffusion blend you want to make, combine equal amounts of lavender, tea tree, and thyme essential oils, and shake well to blend. Store the bottle in a cool, dark place between uses. Diffuse this blend during cold and flu season, or whenever someone in your home is starting to feel under the weather.

INVIGORATING BLACK PEPPER-BERGAMOT BATH

MAKES 1 TREATMENT

Black pepper essential oil is an excellent overall tonic, aiding spleen and colon function while putting its antiseptic property to work keeping colds, flu, and even mental and emotional malaise at bay. Bergamot also helps keep germs at bay while lifting the spirits.

1 tablespoon carrier oil

6 drops black pepper essential oil

6 drops bergamot essential oil

1. In a small glass bowl, add the carrier oil along with the black pepper and bergamot essential oils, and stir to combine.
2. Draw a warm bath and add the entire treatment to the running water.
3. Soak for at least 15 minutes. Use caution when getting out of the bathtub, as it may be slippery.
4. Enjoy this bath anytime illness is going around or whenever you feel like taking a few moments to invest in your health.

Indigestion

Also known as dyspepsia, indigestion causes pressure and discomfort in the upper abdominal area, often resulting in symptoms such as bloating, belching, and nausea. Indigestion may occur shortly after eating, and it is sometimes mistaken for heartburn. Overeating, consuming spicy, fried, or greasy foods, and drinking alcohol with meals can contribute to the problem. Seek medical attention if indigestion is frequent, as an underlying medical condition could be to blame.

INHALE ANISEED

Aniseed essential oil is an excellent remedy for many types of digestive upset, including nausea, vomiting, and general indigestion. Diffuse 1 or 2 drops of aniseed essential oil, or directly inhale it from the bottle. People who have sensitive skin should avoid contact, as dermatitis can occur. Additionally, the essential oil should not be taken internally.

Infection

Swelling, redness, pain, heat, and the presence of pus are among the most prominent infection symptoms. Small, localized infections typically respond well to treatment with essential oils; systemic infections or large infected wounds are considered medical emergencies and require a doctor's intervention.

NEAT CLOVE TREATMENT

Clove essential oil is a powerful antibacterial, antiviral, and antifungal agent. Besides addressing the infection, it numbs pain. Use the smallest amount of clove essential oil possible to treat each infection, and apply it neat. Repeat this treatment every 2 to 3 hours as needed. If you have sensitive skin, dilute clove essential oil with an equal amount of a carrier oil.

NEAT BASIL TREATMENT

Basil essential oil has antibacterial and antiviral properties that make it effective against a wide range of infections. Consider alternating it with clove essential oil to conduct a two-pronged attack on infection. Like clove essential oil, basil essential oil may be applied neat, using the smallest amount needed to treat the area. Repeat this treatment every 2 to 3 hours as needed. Dilute basil essential oil with an equal amount of a carrier oil if you have sensitive skin.

Basil essential oil has been clinically proven to inhibit antibiotic-resistant bacteria. According to a study published in the Journal of Microbiological Methods, basil was able to inhibit bacterial growth of staphylococcus, enterococcus, and pseudomonas bacteria even though these bacteria are resistant to antibiotics.

Inflammation

Inflammation is the body's way of protecting itself from infection. In some diseases such as arthritis, this defense system triggers an immune response when no threat of infection exists, causing pain and swelling. If essential oils do not bring relief, see your doctor.

NEAT BASIL TREATMENT

Basil essential oil is both an anti-inflammatory and antispasmodic, making it an excellent muscle relaxant. When muscles are tired, inflamed, or cramping, basil essential oil promotes rapid relaxation. If you are sensitive to basil or have sensitive skin, dilute the basil essential oil to as low as 1 part essential oil to 4 parts carrier oil. Massage it into the affected area, then relax comfortably. Taking a hot bath or shower before application will intensify the effect.

THYME MASSAGE

MAKES 1 TREATMENT

Thyme essential oil is high in carvacrol, which is a type of phenol that works as a natural anti-inflammatory. This treatment can easily be doubled or tripled for use on large areas of inflamed tissue.

1 tablespoon carrier oil
6 drops thyme essential oil

1. In a small glass bowl, add the carrier oil and thyme essential oil, and stir to combine.
2. Using your fingertips, apply the blend to the affected area, and massage it into the skin.
3. Repeat this treatment up to 3 times a day until the inflammation subsides.

Ingrown Hair

An ingrown hair isn't a serious problem, but it can be embarrassing and irritating. An ingrown hair forms when a hair curls around itself and grows back into the skin rather than rising up from it as it normally would. Ingrown hairs are easily treated at home, and medical intervention is rarely necessary.

REDUCE RISK WITH TEA TREE

Tea tree essential oil prevents infection from developing and can reduce the number of ingrown hairs that develop in a specific area. It penetrates the skin's surface, helping keep bacteria, such as that from your razor blade, out. Add 10 drops to 1 ounce of tea tree essential oil to your regular body lotion, mixing well, and apply it prior to shaving. You can also add 3 or 4 drops of tea tree essential oil to your shaving cream or gel before application.

LAVENDER-CHAMOMILE SUGAR SCRUB

MAKES 1 TREATMENT

Treat existing ingrown hairs by exfoliating. This process removes the dry, dead skin on top, releasing the trapped hairs and encouraging them to grow in the correct direction. The lavender and Roman chamomile essential oils in this treatment help ease inflammation, and the tea tree essential oil addresses infection. This sugar scrub is also great for exfoliating and moisturizing rough, dry skin. The treatment works well with either Roman or German chamomile.

1 tablespoon carrier oil
3 drops lavender essential oil
3 drops Roman chamomile essential oil
3 drops tea tree essential oil
¼ cup granulated sugar

1. In a small glass bowl, add the carrier oil along with the lavender, Roman chamomile, and tea tree essential oils, and stir to combine.
2. Add the sugar to the oils, and stir to combine.
3. Using your fingertips or a washcloth, apply the sugar scrub to moist skin, and rub with light pressure in circular motions.
4. Rinse and pat the skin dry.
5. Repeat this treatment once every other day until symptoms subside, or continue treatment every other day as a preventive measure.

Insect Repellent

Mosquitoes, gnats, chiggers, and other bugs sometimes carry diseases, and their bites are painful and itchy. These natural insect repellents are excellent alternatives to chemical-laden sprays and creams sold commercially.

CITRONELLA SPRAY

MAKES 24 TREATMENTS

Most insects are repelled by citronella; it is such an effective insect repellent that it is used in a number of commercially available products.

4 ounces water
24 drops citronella essential oil

1. In a dark-colored glass bottle fitted with a spray top, add the water and citronella essential oil, and shake to combine.
2. Spray exposed skin and clothing before going outside.
3. Repeat this treatment as needed, avoiding the eye area. Shake the bottle before each use.

GERANIUM-PATCHOULI SPRITZ

MAKES 24 TREATMENTS

Geranium essential oil contains geraniol, which many manufacturers use in the production of natural insect repellents. Patchouli essential oil has a time-honored history as an effective insect repellent, and it lends a lovely fragrance to this delightful insect repellent.

4 ounces water
24 drops geranium essential oil
24 drops patchouli essential oil

1. In a dark-colored glass bottle fitted with a spray top, add the water along with the geranium and patchouli essential oils, and shake well to blend.
2. Spray exposed skin and clothing before going outside.
3. Repeat this treatment as needed, avoiding the eye area. Shake the bottle before each use.

Insomnia

Insomnia is characterized by difficulty falling asleep or staying asleep. Some sufferers wake often during the night and have difficulty going back to sleep, some have trouble falling asleep even though they are tired, and some wake up early in the morning and can't get back to sleep. Almost all insomnia sufferers are chronically exhausted. If your insomnia does not respond to natural treatments, visit your doctor to rule out an underlying medical condition.

NEROLI-SPIKENARD BEDTIME MASSAGE

MAKES 12 TREATMENTS

Both neroli and spikenard essential oils have strong sedative properties, and are ideal for inclusion in bedtime routines, particularly for those who have a tough time falling or staying asleep. For extra benefits from this treatment, be sure that your bedroom is quiet and dark; watching TV or using electronics right before bed can disrupt sleep.

3 ounces carrier oil
24 drops neroli essential oil
12 drops spikenard essential oil

1. In a dark-colored glass bottle, add the carrier oil along with the neroli and spikenard essential oils, and shake well to blend.
2. Using your fingertips, apply 1 tablespoon of the blend to the body just before getting into bed.
3. Repeat this treatment once a day at bedtime until normal sleeping patterns resume.

LAVENDER-PETITGRAIN BATH OIL

MAKES 1 TREATMENT

Lavender essential oil is such an effective natural sleep aid that it is included in numerous commercial preparations intended to promote relaxation and restful sleep. Petitgrain essential oil is used less often, but it is an effective relaxant nonetheless. Light the bathroom with a candle or two instead of leaving the electric lights on, and you'll find this bath even more effective. Vetiver essential oil may be used instead of petitgrain essential oil, if preferred.

1 tablespoon carrier oil
10 drops lavender essential oil
5 drops petitgrain essential oil

1. In a small glass bowl, add the carrier oil along with the lavender and petitgrain essential oils, and stir to combine.
2. Draw a warm bath and add the entire treatment to the running water.
3. Soak for at least 15 minutes. Use caution when getting out of the bathtub, as it may be slippery.
4. Repeat this treatment once a day at bedtime until normal sleeping patterns resume.

Achieve rest naturally. Lavender has been proven to outperform common pharmaceuticals in decreasing anxiety, enhancing relaxation, and promoting sleep, according to a 1988 study published in the International Journal of Aromatherapy. Just sprinkling a few drops on your pillowcase will promote deep, restful sleep.

Intestinal Parasites

Intestinal parasites are organisms that live in the digestive tract, causing symptoms such as bloating and intestinal pain, excess flatulence, pale skin, tiredness, and blood or mucus in the stool. In many cases, worms or their eggs may be seen in bowel movements. See a doctor if treatment with essential oils does not produce the desired effect.

NIAOULI-EUCALYPTUS MASSAGE

MAKES 1 TREATMENT

Eucalyptus, lemon, niaouli, and Roman chamomile essential oils come together to create a synergistic blend that the body absorbs to ward off intestinal parasites. This treatment is particularly effective after a warm bath. Eating food prepared with plenty of garlic proves helpful during treatment, as well. This remedy is effective for children; adults should use a double dose.

2 tablespoons carrier oil
8 drops eucalyptus essential oil
8 drops lavender essential oil
8 drops niaouli essential oil
8 drops Roman chamomile essential oil

1. In a small glass bowl, add the carrier oil along with the eucalyptus, lavender, niaouli, and Roman chamomile essential oils, and stir to combine.
2. Using your fingertips, apply the entire treatment to the abdomen, and massage it gently into the skin.
3. Repeat this treatment 2 times a day for 3 days.

CINNAMON-THYME COMPRESS

MAKES 1 TREATMENT

Cinnamon, fennel, and thyme essential oils aid in expelling parasites; using a hot compress helps propel the essential oils into the abdomen while easing the gas, cramping, and bloating that so often accompany infestation. This remedy is intended for children; adults should double the dose.

2 tablespoons carrier oil
5 drops cinnamon essential oil
5 drops fennel essential oil
5 drops thyme essential oil
1 pint hot water

1. In a small glass bowl, add the carrier oil along with the cinnamon, fennel, and thyme essential oils, and stir to combine.
2. Using your fingertips, apply the entire treatment to the abdomen, and massage it into the skin.
3. In a medium glass bowl, add the hot water.

4. Submerge a towel in the water, wring it out, and apply the compress to the affected area. Layer plastic wrap on top of the compress to keep the essential oil vapors from evaporating. Leave the compress in place until it cools to body temperature.

5. Repeat this treatment 2 times a day for 3 days.

Jock Itch

Jock itch is caused by fungal growth in or on the groin's top layer of skin. Itching, burning, and a rash are usually present, and heat or tight clothing can exacerbate symptoms. Jock itch is extremely contagious, so it's important that you avoid contact with items others will touch or use. While essential oils provide fast relief in most cases, those with underlying infections may require medical intervention.

TEA TREE SPRAY

MAKES 24 TREATMENTS

Tea tree essential oil is the ideal weapon in your arsenal against jock itch, thanks to its powerful antifungal action.

4 ounces water
48 drops tea tree essential oil

1. In a dark-colored glass bottle fitted with a spray top, add the water and tea tree essential oil, and shake well to blend.
2. Spray the affected area generously after showering. Allow the area to dry before dressing.
3. Repeat this treatment up to 4 times a day until symptoms subside. Shake the bottle before each use.

EUCALYPTUS-TEA TREE BALM

MAKES 12 TREATMENTS

Eucalyptus, lavender, and tea tree essential oils come together to heal the sore, cracked skin that sometimes accompanies jock itch. At the same time, their antifungal action addresses the fungal infection that causes the ailment.

4 tablespoons carrier oil
24 drops eucalyptus essential oil
24 drops lavender essential oil
24 drops tea tree essential oil

1. In a dark-colored glass bottle, add the carrier oil along with the eucalyptus, lavender, and tea tree essential oils, and shake well to blend.
2. Using your fingertips, apply 1 teaspoon to the affected area.
3. Repeat this treatment once a day at bedtime until the jock itch has subsided.

Keratosis Pilaris

Often referred to simply as "chicken skin," keratosis pilaris is a skin condition characterized by small red, purple, or white bumps on the skin, usually on the back sides of the upper arms and thighs. In many cases, itching and dry skin accompany the bumps, which are usually a cosmetic problem rather than a medical one. Seek medical attention if severe redness, inflammation, or an infection is present.

GERANIUM-CITRUS SOAK

MAKES 1 TREATMENT

Moisturizing well is vital to reducing the appearance of keratosis pilaris. Moisturize your skin before using any type of scrub, as it will help remove the sebum plugs from pores and follicles. Geranium essential oil addresses inflammation and improves skin tone, and the lemon and tangerine essential oils aid in softening the skin prior to exfoliation. Use bergamot, lime, or orange essential oils to replace the lemon or tangerine, if desired.

1 tablespoon carrier oil
6 drops geranium essential oil
6 drops lemon essential oil
6 drops tangerine essential oil

1. In a small glass bowl, add the carrier oil along with the geranium, lemon, and tangerine essential oils, and stir well to combine.
2. Draw a warm bath and add the entire treatment to the running water.
3. Soak for at least 15 minutes.
4. Using a loofa or other natural fiber, exfoliate after soaking.
5. Shower to remove the dead skin. Use caution when standing in the bathtub, as it may be slippery.
6. Repeat this treatment once a day until symptoms subside, or continue treatment as a preventive measure.

MANDARIN-TAGETES SCRUB

MAKES 1 TREATMENT

The mandarin essential oil aids in moisturizing and soothing the skin during the exfoliation process. Tagetes essential oil has strong antimicrobial properties that make it ideal for inclusion in this scrub. If you have none on hand, use tea tree essential oil in its place. Avoid sun exposure for at least 12 hours after this treatment, as both tagetes and mandarin essential oils cause photosensitivity.

2 tablespoons carrier oil

4 drops mandarin essential oil

2 drops tagetes essential oil

½ cup granulated sugar

1. In a small glass bowl, add the carrier oil along with the mandarin and tagetes essential oils, and stir to combine.
2. Add the sugar to the oils, and stir to combine.
3. Draw a warm bath and soak for at least 15 minutes.
4. Using your fingertips or a washcloth, apply the scrub to the affected area, and massage with medium to firm pressure in circular motions, then rinse. Use caution when getting out of the bathtub, as it may be slippery.
5. Repeat this treatment every 3 to 4 days until the keratosis pilaris has subsided.

Knee Pain

Knee pain may be sharp or dull; it may be chronic, or it may occur as the result of an injury. Some types of knee pain respond very well to treatment with essential oils; others require surgical intervention. If your knee pain is the result of an injury and is severe, or if your knee is not capable of bearing weight, you should seek emergency treatment. The longer you let a knee injury go, the more complicated it may be for doctors to repair the joint's internal structures.

The knee isn't just a hinge. It is a very complicated mechanism, with four bones, four ligaments for stability, and numerous tendons that facilitate leg motion. Cartilage provides some cushioning, and fluid-filled sacs called bursas provide additional cushioning between the knee's bones. When any of these structures is compromised, your knee's ability to bear your weight and provide motility can be severely reduced.

MASSAGE WITH PINE BLEND

Pine essential oil is an excellent antirheumatic agent that penetrates deep into tissue; it also helps promote circulation, which helps injured tissue heal faster. Pine essential oil is strong and should be diluted. In a dark-colored glass bottle large enough to hold the amount you want to make, dilute the essential oil with equal amounts of a carrier oil before using it as a pain reliever. Apply the treatment with your fingertips, massaging it into the skin to encourage absorption. Repeat this treatment as needed.

PEPPERMINT-EUCALYPTUS LINIMENT

MAKES 24 TREATMENTS

Peppermint and eucalyptus essential oils have analgesic, anesthetic, and anti-inflammatory properties that make them ideal for treating sore joints.

4 ounces carrier oil
24 drops peppermint essential oil
24 drops eucalyptus essential oil

1. In a dark-colored glass bottle, add the carrier oil along with the peppermint and eucalyptus essential oils, and shake well to blend.
2. Using your fingertips, apply 1 teaspoon of the blend to the affected area, and massage it into the skin.
3. Repeat this treatment once a day until the knee pain subsides. Store the bottle in a cool, dark place between uses.

Laryngitis

Laryngitis is inflammation of the larynx or voice box, and causes your voice to become hoarse or raspy. Often caused by a cold or the flu, and sometimes a complication of acid reflux or irritation caused by allergies, laryngitis typically comes on quickly and lasts for two weeks or less. See your doctor if the condition worsens or if symptoms last longer than two weeks.

CAJEPUT STEAM TREATMENT

MAKES 1 TREATMENT

Cajeput essential oil is an excellent natural analgesic that helps stop pain associated with laryngitis. Use it in a vapor treatment to deliver the essential oil directly to the affected area. You may also diffuse it or put a few drops in a hot bath.

3 cups hot water
6 drops cajeput essential oil

1. In a large shallow glass bowl, add the hot water and cajeput essential oil, and stir to combine.
2. Sit comfortably, tenting your head with a towel over the bowl, and breathe deeply for several minutes, emerging for fresh air as needed.
3. Repeat this treatment every 2 to 3 hours as needed until symptoms subside.

SOOTHING LEMON GARGLE

MAKES 1 TREATMENT

Lemon and niaouli essential oils have anti-inflammatory, antiseptic, and analgesic properties that make them ideal for easing the pain and inflammation that accompany laryngitis.

1 ounce warm water

2 drops lemon essential oil

2 drops niaouli essential oil

1. In a small drinking glass, add the warm water along with the lemon and niaouli essential oils, and stir to combine.
2. Gargle with the entire blend for at least 30 seconds. Do not swallow the blend.
3. Repeat this treatment every 2 to 3 hours as needed until symptoms subside.

Leg Cramps

Leg cramps can accompany dehydration, overtired muscles, obesity, and pregnancy; some are caused by low calcium intake. Minor leg cramps respond well to stretching, exercise, and treatment with essential oils as well as an iron-rich diet to prevent anemia. Leg cramps that don't go away, or are accompanied by swelling and a general inability to walk properly need to be addressed by a physician.

ANTI-CRAMPING MASSAGE OIL

MAKES 8 TREATMENTS

Marjoram, rosemary, hyssop, and lavender essential oils come together in this treatment, preventing the muscle spasms that lead to leg cramps, particularly at night. Make sure your muscles are warm before applying this treatment.

4 ounces carrier oil

40 drops marjoram essential oil

40 drops rosemary essential oil

20 drops hyssop essential oil

20 drops lavender essential oil

1. In a dark-colored glass bottle, add the carrier oil along with the marjoram, rosemary, hyssop, and lavender essential oils, and shake well to blend.
2. Using your fingertips, apply ½ tablespoon of the blend to each leg before bed, and massage it in an upward direction.
3. Massage your feet last, then put on socks to keep your feet warm.
4. Repeat this treatment once a day at bedtime for at least 2 weeks.

GERANIUM-EVENING PRIMROSE RUB

MAKES 1 TREATMENT

Geranium and evening primrose oil have antispasmodic and anti-inflammatory properties that make them ideal for stopping cramps in progress. Use rose geranium essential oil if you have no geranium essential oil on hand.

1 teaspoon evening primrose essential oil
4 drops geranium essential oil

1. Using your fingertips, apply the evening primrose essential oil to the affected area, followed by the geranium essential oil.
2. Massage vigorously until the cramping stops.
3. Repeat this treatment up to 3 times a day as needed.

Lice

A lice infestation can quickly spread. Symptoms include itching and tiny red bites; nits, or louse eggs, can be seen clinging to the hair. Adult lice and nymphs may be difficult to spot. If one of your family members has head lice, treat everyone. Seek medical intervention if essential oils do not make a difference.

GERANIUM SHAMPOO

Add geranium or rose geranium essential oil to natural shampoo to effectively kill adult and nymph lice; you will need to remove nits separately to keep them from hatching. In a glass bottle or a small glass bowl, combine 4 ounces of natural shampoo with 40 drops of geranium or rose geranium essential oil, and shake or stir to combine. Apply the shampoo to the entire head, scrubbing vigorously. Leave the shampoo in place for 10 minutes, taking care not to get suds in the eyes. Rinse and follow up with a conditioner. Remove the nits with a fine-tooth comb.

NEAT TEA TREE TREATMENT

Tea tree essential oil kills adult lice and nymphs. Be sure to check for nits separately and remove them with a fine-toothed comb. Apply as much tea tree essential oil as needed to the scalp and leave it in place for 40 minutes, then shampoo and condition the hair. Check for lice every few days, and repeat this treatment until they have been eradicated.

Low Energy

There are many reasons you may feel less than energetic; perhaps your schedule induces fatigue, or it could be that stress is starting to erode feelings of overall well-being. Essential oils are ideal for enhancing energy naturally. Use a variety of different oils regularly for the best possible outcome.

PEPPERMINT NECK MASSAGE

Peppermint essential oil balances and reinvigorates by stimulating the body and mind alike. This cooling neck massage is quick and easy to do anywhere. Drip 4 drops of peppermint essential oil onto the palm of your dominant hand and swipe your hand across the back of your neck just beneath your hairline. Massage the back of the neck for at least 2 minutes, then work your way up the back of your head toward your crown, stopping about halfway up. Repeat this treatment hourly, if needed.

PEPPERMINT-ROSEMARY INHALATION

MAKES 1 TREATMENT

Both peppermint and rosemary essential oils impart feelings of energy and alertness. When combined, they emit an irresistible fragrance that is certain to reinvigorate you. In a small glass bowl, combine 4 drops of peppermint essential oil and 4 drops of rosemary essential oil, and stir to combine. Add the essential oils to an aromatherapy pendant or diffuser, according to the manufacturer's directions. Inhale deeply to increase energy and alertness.

Low Testosterone Support

Men suffering from low testosterone often feel fatigued, depressed, and weak; in addition, lack of libido and erectile dysfunction often accompany low testosterone. If you notice no improvement after three weeks of essential oils treatments, see your doctor.

JASMINE AROMATHERAPY

Jasmine essential oil soothes and calms while acting as a powerful aphrodisiac. Diffuse the oil in your bedroom and in areas where you tend to spend the most time, carry an aromatherapy pendant you can inhale from throughout the day, or create a simple massage oil with 1 tablespoon of carrier oil and 4 drops of jasmine essential oil.

YLANG-YLANG MASSAGE OIL

MAKES 8 TREATMENTS

Ylang-ylang essential oil has long been revered for its effectiveness as an aphrodisiac, and it promotes feelings of peaceful euphoria and contented relaxation. Black pepper essential oil is also an aphrodisiac; it increases circulation while toning smooth muscles, including those involved in the erectile process. You can also use 1 tablespoon of this blend in a warm bath.

4 ounces carrier oil
20 drops ylang-ylang essential oil
20 drops black pepper essential oil

1. In a dark-colored glass bottle, add the carrier oil along with the ylang-ylang and black pepper essential oils, and shake well to blend.
2. Using your fingertips, apply 1 tablespoon of the blend to the arms, legs, back, chest, and abdomen, and massage it into the skin.
3. Repeat this treatment once a day at bedtime as needed. Store the bottle in a cool, dark place between uses.

Lupus

Lupus is an autoimmune disease that occurs when the immune system attacks the body's tissues, leading to swelling, inflammation, fever, fatigue, and a rash. Brain fog is often present, and patients often suffer from depression. Essential oils can help bring comfort and decrease symptoms. Use them with your caregiver's approval.

LEMON VERBENA BATH OIL

MAKES 8 TREATMENTS

Lemon verbena essential oil stimulates the internal organs and relaxes the body and mind. You may also benefit by diffusing lemon verbena essential oil in the area where you spend the most time. Avoid sun exposure for at least 12 hours after using this treatment, as lemon verbena essential oil can cause photosensitivity.

4 ounces carrier oil
20 drops lemon verbena essential oil

1. In a dark-colored glass bottle, add the carrier oil and lemon verbena essential oil, and shake well to blend.
2. Draw a warm bath and add 1 tablespoon of the blend to the running water.
3. Soak for at least 15 minutes, then rinse. Use caution when getting out of the bathtub, as it may be slippery.
4. Repeat this treatment once a day as needed. Store the bottle in a cool, dark place between uses.

LIME MASSAGE OIL

MAKES 1 TREATMENT

Lime essential oil does wonders for blue moods, lifting mental fog and lightening one's outlook on life. In addition, it is a powerful anti-inflammatory and immune support agent, relieving muscle and joint pain while revitalizing the body. You may also use this treatment in a bath by adding the full amount to a tubful of warm water and soaking for 15 minutes.

1 tablespoon carrier oil
6 drops lime essential oil

1. In a small glass bowl, add the carrier oil and lime essential oil, and stir to combine.
2. Using your fingertips, apply the blend to the affected area, and massage it into the skin.
3. Repeat this treatment once a day at bedtime.

Lyme Disease

Lyme disease is a tick-borne infection carried by deer ticks and western black-legged ticks. Remove ticks as soon as you spot them, as it normally takes at least 36 hours for an infected tick to spread Lyme disease to its host. Symptoms include sore joints and muscles, fever, headache, poor memory, flu-like symptoms, and a round, red rash; they can appear between three days and one month from the time of the bite. See your doctor, and support your immune system with essential oils.

Lyme disease can cause life-long problems if left untreated. The skin, joints, heart, and nervous system can be damaged by a prolonged Lyme disease infection; facial paralysis, pain similar to arthritis, and numbness and tingling in the back, feet, and hands are common symptoms of untreated Lyme disease. Pain and other long-term problems can recur even months or years after the original tick bite.

DIFFUSE ROSEMARY

Rosemary essential oil has been proven to help increase mental clarity and improve retention, making it the ideal tool for combating the mental fog that often accompanies Lyme disease. It also aids in eliminating fatigue and headaches, so make it a go-to treatment for handling symptoms. Diffuse rosemary essential oil in areas where you spend time, enjoy it in an aromatherapy pendant, or inhale the scent directly from the bottle as needed. Rosemary essential oil is not recommended for those with epilepsy or hypertension, or who are pregnant.

SOOTHING IMMUNE-BOOSTER BATH

MAKES 1 TREATMENT

Lavender, lemon, and tea tree essential oils combine to help support the immune system while you are recovering from Lyme disease. They are particularly helpful in alleviating flu-like symptoms.

1 tablespoon carrier oil
8 drops tea tree essential oil
6 drops lavender essential oil
2 drops lemon essential oil

1. In a small glass bowl, add the carrier oil along with the tea tree, lavender, and lemon essential oils, and stir well to combine.
2. Draw a warm bath and add the entire treatment to the running water.
3. Soak for at least 15 minutes. Use caution when getting out of the bathtub, as it may be slippery.
4. Repeat this treatment once a day until symptoms subside.

Menopause

Night sweats and difficulty sleeping, hot flashes, irritability, and irregular periods are among the chief symptoms of menopause. Essential oils offer relief from many of these symptoms, making it possible for many sufferers to avoid chemical-based treatments altogether. Be sure to continue preventive care, including breast cancer screening, during this time.

DIFFUSE CLARY SAGE

Clary sage essential oil is highly regarded for its ability to ease stress, anxiety, irritability, and the feelings of discomfort that accompany menopause. Diffuse clary sage essential oil in the area where you spend the most time, or carry it with you in an aromatherapy pendant to reap its rewards. You can also add 5 or 6 drops to a warm bath before bed to help ease symptoms.

CLARY SAGE-GERANIUM MASSAGE OIL

MAKES 8 TREATMENTS

Clary sage and geranium essential oils come together in this delightful massage oil, easing tension, alleviating stress, and addressing feelings of depression. You may also use this treatment in a bath by adding 1 tablespoon of the blend to a tubful of warm water and soaking for 15 minutes. The lavender in this blend helps promote restful sleep; eliminate it if you use this massage oil anytime other than before bed.

4 ounces carrier oil
16 drops clary sage essential oil
16 drops geranium essential oil
16 drops lavender essential oil

1. In a dark-colored glass bottle, add the carrier oil along with the clary sage, geranium, and lavender essential oils, and shake well to blend.
2. Using your fingertips, apply 1 tablespoon of the blend to the arms, legs, chest, back, and abdomen, and massage it into the skin.
3. Repeat this treatment 3 times a day.

Mental Alertness

Absentmindedness, drowsiness, and a lack of motivation can negatively impact your life. Maintain a lively state of attentiveness, keep your memory in good shape, and improve your reflexes by pairing essential oils with an active lifestyle and good nutrition. If a lack of mental alertness plagues you daily, see your doctor to rule out an underlying medical condition.

INHALE ROSEMARY

Rosemary essential oil has been proven to facilitate mental clarity and aid in memory retention. It is ideal for use when working, studying, or practicing an instrument, and its aroma is a pleasant one that will leave your indoor environment smelling fantastic. Hyssop essential oil has similar effects and may be used in place of rosemary essential oil. You may use any inhalation method: inhale its scent directly from the bottle; diffuse rosemary essential oil in the area where you spend the most time, or place some in an aromatherapy pendant. You can also add 1 to 3 drops of rosemary essential oil to your bath or to a washcloth placed on the floor of your shower.

STIMULATING CITRUS BATH

MAKES 1 TREATMENT

Lemon and tangerine essential oils come together to eliminate drowsiness, sharpen focus, and create a sense of total well-being. This is also an excellent blend to use as an all-purpose air freshener or diffuser in your home or office, or place some in an aroma-therapy pendant.

3 drops lemon essential oil
3 drops tangerine essential oil

1. In a small glass bowl, add the lemon and tangerine essential oils, and stir to combine.
2. Draw a warm bath and add 2 or 3 drops of the blend to the running water.
3. Soak for at least 15 minutes. Use caution when getting out of the bathtub, as it may be slippery.
4. Repeat this treatment once a day as needed.

Mental Health

Everyone has ups and downs; in fact an estimated 22 percent of Americans are affected by mental health issues. Consider using essential oils to bolster your mental well-being, whether you take prescriptions or not.

DIFFUSE ROSEWOOD

Rosewood essential oil balances mind and body alike, lifting the spirits, helping with headaches, and boosting the immune system. Diffuse 3 to 5 drops of rosewood essential oil in the area where you spend the most time, and consider adding 1 or 2 drops in an aromatherapy pendant to take advantage of the essential oil's benefits throughout the day. Rosewood essential oil is also an aid to effective meditation.

ROSEMARY-SAGE BALANCING TREATMENT

MAKES 1 TREATMENT

Rosemary and sage combine to calm the nerves, alleviate feelings of depression, and improve overall mental function. This is an outstanding blend to diffuse when working; it sharpens focus and facilitates a positive outlook. In a small glass bowl, blend 3 drops of rosemary essential oil with 3 drops of sage essential oil, and diffuse the blend. You may also add 1 or 2 drops to your bath or to a washcloth placed on the floor of your shower.

Stay calm and alert with rosemary. In a study conducted at the University of Miami School of Medicine, participants discovered they were able to complete math computations rapidly and with accuracy when using rosemary essential oil. It has been shown to increase relaxation and alertness while alleviating anxiety.

Migraine

Often triggered by food or outside stimuli, migraines are severe headaches that tend to be accompanied by light sensitivity, nausea, vomiting, blurred vision, or a migraine aura—with visual hallucinations such as wavy lines, bright flashing lights, or blind spots. Migraines often respond well to treatment with essential oils; if they are frequent and unresponsive, see your doctor to rule out an underlying disease.

INHALE LEMON

Lemon essential oil helps reduce blood pressure and improve circulation, and it is renowned for its ability to soothe migraine symptoms and induce a relaxed but alert mental state. You may directly inhale this essential oil, or you may choose to diffuse it or place it in an aromatherapy pendant. You can also add 1 to 3 drops to your bath or to a washcloth placed on the floor of your shower. Lemon essential oil can be used alone or in concert with other therapies.

SOOTHING CORIANDER MASSAGE

MAKES 1 TREATMENT

Coriander is a strong analgesic that also acts against nausea. Because it can have a sensitizing effect on some individuals, it is very important that you conduct a patch test prior to using this oil.

1 tablespoon carrier oil
8 drops coriander essential oil

1. In a small glass bowl, add the carrier oil and coriander essential oil, and stir to combine.
2. Using your fingertips, apply the blend to the arms, legs, abdomen, back, and chest, and massage it into the skin.
3. Repeat this treatment as needed to alleviate migraine symptoms, either alone or in concert with other therapies.

Morning Sickness

Morning sickness typically occurs during the first trimester of pregnancy, and is marked by nausea and vomiting. Acupressure, avoiding triggers such as smells and foods that tend to lead to nausea, and eating bland foods can help, as can treatment with essential oils. Talk to your caregiver if morning sickness is severe and dehydration or weight loss is occurring. Hospitalization is occasionally required in the worst cases.

DIFFUSE GINGER

Ginger essential oil is safe for use during early pregnancy and is among the best essential oils for eliminating nausea. Diffuse it in the area where you spend the most time, and put 1 drop of it on your pillowcase each night. You may also use it in an aromatherapy pendant or simply put a few drops on a cotton ball and keep it nearby.

SPEARMINT VAPORS

MAKES 1 TREATMENT

Spearmint essential oil is safe for inhalation during early pregnancy, and its aroma helps keep queasiness at bay.

8 cups boiling water
12 drops spearmint essential oil

1. In a shallow glass bowl, add the boiling water and spearmint essential oil, and stir to combine.
2. Place the bowl near your bed at bed time. The scent will gently waft throughout your bedroom and help promote a calm stomach.
3. Repeat this treatment for 3 nights in a row; by the third morning, you should not feel nausea on awakening.

Motion Sickness

Nausea, sometimes accompanied by vomiting, is the chief symptom of motion sickness, which occurs when the eyes and inner ears send conflicting or unexpected messages to the brain, throwing your sense of balance off. Stop the motion if you can, and use these simple remedies to feel better fast.

GINGER TRAVEL THERAPY

MAKES 24 TREATMENTS

Ginger essential oil is among the best available remedies for motion sickness. Use this travel therapy to help children, pets, and others cope with car travel, or spritz it on your clothing before air travel.

4 ounces water
24 drops ginger essential oil

1. In a dark-colored glass bottle fitted with a spray top, combine the water and ginger essential oil, and shake well to blend.
2. Spray the blend in your car's interior.
3. Repeat this treatment as needed. Shake the bottle before each use.

Ease nausea naturally with ginger. One of the worst forms of motion sickness, seasickness can be difficult to treat. According to the University of Maryland Medical Center, in a study of sailors prone to seasickness, ginger was proven to ease symptoms of cold sweating and vomiting, while those given a placebo reported no relief.

GRAPEFRUIT SMELLING SALTS

MAKES 1 TREATMENT

Grapefruit essential oil uplifts the spirits, promotes feelings of total well-being, and helps address the nausea and discomfort that characterize motion sickness. This simple remedy is one you can use any time without disturbing others.

1 tablespoon sea salt
6 drops grapefruit essential oil

1. In a dark-colored glass bottle, add the salt and grapefruit essential oil, and shake well to blend.
2. Inhale from the bottle.
3. Repeat this treatment as needed. Refresh the smelling salt periodically by adding 3 or 4 drops of grapefruit essential oil.

Mud Fever

Also known as leptospirosis, canefield fever, field fever, or seven-day fever, mud fever is a bacterial disease with symptoms that include headache, vomiting, diarrhea, high fever, jaundice, chills, and muscle aches. Seek medical attention immediately if you believe you have mud fever, as serious complications can occur if the disease is left untreated. Use essential oils to reduce discomfort throughout the course of treatment.

LEMON COMPRESS

MAKES 1 TREATMENT

Lemon essential oil is effective in combating nausea and alleviating headaches, making it an excellent tool for use in alleviating the symptoms that accompany mud fever. This compress aids in cooling fever and may be used as frequently as desired.

6 drops carrier oil
3 drops lemon essential oil
1 pint cold water

1. In a small glass bowl, add the carrier oil and lemon essential oil, and stir to combine.
2. Using your fingertips, apply the blend to the temples and forehead, and massage it into the skin.
3. In a medium bowl, add the cold water.
4. Submerge a towel in the water, wring it out, and apply the compress to the affected area. Leave the compress in place until it warms to body temperature.
5. Reapply compresses until the water in the bowl loses its chill.
6. Repeat this treatment as needed.

NIAOULI BATH OIL

MAKES 1 TREATMENT

Niaouli essential oil is a strong decongestant that fortifies the immune system and helps alleviate pain. With this bath treatment, you benefit by absorption and inhalation. Use tea tree essential oil if you do not have niaouli essential oil available.

1 tablespoon carrier oil
8 drops niaouli essential oil

1. In a small glass bowl, add the carrier oil and niaouli essential oil, and stir to combine.
2. Draw a warm bath and add the entire treatment to the running water.
3. Soak for at least 15 minutes. Use caution when getting out of the bathtub, as it may be slippery.
4. Repeat this treatment up to 3 times a day while recuperating.

Multiple Sclerosis

Multiple sclerosis (MS) affects the brain and spinal cord. In the disease's early stages, symptoms include weakness, numbness, tingling, and blurred vision, along with muscle stiffness, urinary problems, and complications with mental processes. MS requires medical intervention; use essential oils to complement therapy with your doctor's approval.

DIFFUSE FRANKINCENSE

Frankincense essential oil calms the mind, soothing worries and promoting deep, even breathing. It also helps with anxiety. Diffuse it regularly in areas where you spend time, and consider keeping some with you in an aromatherapy pendant. Because it is good for skin and for use as a general physical tonic, 1 to 3 drops of frankincense essential oil may also be enjoyed in a massage oil, in the bath, or on a washcloth placed on the floor of your shower.

JASMINE-NEROLI MASSAGE OIL

MAKES 8 TREATMENTS

Neroli and jasmine essential oils offer support by alleviating chronic stress, anxiety, depression, and fear. They also aid in relaxation, soothing headaches, and easing feelings of vertigo, which by turn may help you feel more comfortable.

4 ounces carrier oil
12 drops jasmine essential oil
12 drops neroli essential oil

1. In a dark-colored glass bottle, add the carrier oil along with the jasmine and neroli essential oils, and shake well to blend.
2. Using your fingertips, apply 1 tablespoon of the blend to the arms, legs, abdomen, back, and chest, and massage it into the skin.
3. Repeat this treatment as needed.

Mumps

Mumps is a highly contagious viral infection that causes pain and swelling of the salivary glands in most cases. Some sufferers feel as though they have a bad cold or sinus infection, and may experience a fever, sore throat, fatigue, nausea, vomiting, and reduced appetite. In rare cases, swollen, painful testicles, severe abdominal pain, severe neck pain with stiffness, and severe headaches are present. If these symptoms arise, seek treatment, as complications may occur.

COOLING ROOM SPRAY

MAKES 24 TREATMENTS

Coriander, lavender, niaouli, and tea tree essential oils come together in this cooling room spray, which helps soothe mumps symptoms and prevent the spread of bacteria.

4 ounces water
10 drops coriander essential oil
10 drops lavender essential oil
10 drops niaouli essential oil
10 drops tea tree essential oil

1. In a dark-colored glass bottle fitted with a spray top, add the water along with the coriander, lavender, niaouli, and tea tree essential oils, and shake well to blend.
2. Spray the blend generously throughout the room where the patient is spending the most time.
3. Repeat this treatment as needed. Shake the bottle before each use.

MUMPS MASSAGE

MAKES 1 TREATMENT

Coriander, lavender, lemon, and tea tree essential oils ease the pain and inflammation that accompanies mumps while also promoting relaxation.

1 tablespoon carrier oil

4 drops coriander essential oil

4 drops lavender essential oil

4 drops lemon essential oil

4 drops tea tree essential oil

1. In a small glass bowl, add the carrier oil along with the coriander, lavender, lemon, and tea tree essential oils, and stir to combine.
2. Using your fingertips, apply the blend to sore areas as well as the abdomen, back of the neck, and temples.
3. Repeat this treatment up to 3 times a day for up to 10 days in a row.

Muscle Aches

Tired, aching muscles are often caused by overwork or strain. Sports trauma often leads to sore muscles, too. Rest, ice or heat, and essential oils are usually enough to provide relief, and muscle aches typically go away after 2 or 3 days. If accompanied by a high fever or other worrisome symptoms, muscle aches may be cause for concern; see your doctor for a diagnosis and treatment.

THYME MASSAGE

MAKES 1 TREATMENT

Thyme essential oil has a penetrating warming quality that makes it ideal for soothing sore muscles. Some can be sensitive to its topical application, so conduct a patch test to determine whether a dilution of equal amounts carrier oil and essential oil will work for you or if you need to increase the amount of carrier oil.

10 drops carrier oil
10 drops thyme essential oil

1. In a small glass bowl, add the carrier oil and thyme essential oil, and stir to combine.
2. Using your fingertips, apply the blend to the affected area, and massage it into the skin.
3. Repeat this treatment as needed during recuperation.

SOOTHING PINE-LAVENDER BATH

MAKES 1 TREATMENT

Pine essential oil is warming, refreshing, and renewing to sore, tired muscles. The lavender essential oil in this blend promotes deep relaxation, helping muscles recuperate faster. This remedy is particularly nice after a long day of physical labor.

1 tablespoon carrier oil
6 drops pine essential oil
4 drops lavender essential oil

1. In a small glass bowl, add the carrier oil along with the pine and lavender essential oils, and stir to combine.
2. Draw a warm bath and add the entire treatment to the running water.
3. Soak for at least 15 minutes. Use caution when getting out of the bathtub, as it may be slippery.
4. Repeat this treatment as needed.

Nail Care

The fingernails are formed of keratin, which is the same substance that forms hair and skin. Instead of using chemical-laden solutions sold commercially, use essential oils to keep your nails strong, healthy, and attractive.

MASSAGE CUTICLES WITH ROSE

Rose essential oil softens, hydrates, and rejuvenates skin while increasing circulation, which in turn may help stimulate healthy nail growth. Use 2 or 3 drops of rose essential oil per hand, gently rubbing the cuticles while enjoying the essential oil's beautiful fragrance. Follow up with a generous dollop of your favorite hand cream. Repeat this treatment as often as you like.

NATURAL NAIL STRENGTHENER

MAKES 24 TREATMENTS

Vitamin E and lavender essential oil come together to help strengthen nails while imparting a natural, healthy glow. If you have no vitamin E oil available, you can extract vitamin E from a capsule by pricking it with a pin and squeezing out as much as you need.

1 teaspoon vitamin E oil
24 drops lavender essential oil

1. In a dark-colored glass bottle, add the vitamin E oil and lavender essential oil, and shake well to blend.
2. Using your fingertips, apply 1 to 3 drops to the nails and cuticles.
3. Repeat this treatment once a day, or as needed.

Nail Fungus

Nail fungus is typically characterized by thickening and yellowing, and usually begins as a single spot of white or yellow under a fingernail or toenail. As the fungus spreads, your nails may begin to crumble, and pain may develop. Treat nail fungus as soon as you notice it to prevent it from becoming a serious problem. See your doctor if essential oils fail to relieve symptoms.

TEA TREE TREATMENT

Tea tree essential oil is a powerful antifungal agent that has the ability to kill nail fungus rapidly. Apply 1 or 2 drops of tea tree essential oil to the affected area, making sure you coat the entire nail, the surrounding skin, and the area beneath the nail's edge. Allow the tea tree oil to penetrate, then cover it with a few drops of a carrier oil. Repeat this treatment up to 3 times a day until symptoms subside.

CLOVE TREATMENT

Clove essential oil is an exceptional antifungal agent. It also stops itching associated with nail fungus. Apply 1 or 2 drops of clove essential oil to the affected area, making sure that you coat the entire nail, the surrounding skin, and the area beneath the nail's edge. Allow the essential oil to penetrate, then cover it with a few drops of carrier oil. Repeat this treatment up to 3 times a day until symptoms subside.

Nasal Polyps

Nasal polyps are teardrop-shaped growths that commonly form in the nose or sinus, often accompanying asthma or allergies. Small nasal polyps usually go unnoticed, but larger ones can block sinus drainage. Surgical intervention is sometimes required, so visit your doctor if natural treatments don't seem to be working.

NEAT FRANKINCENSE TREATMENT

Frankincense essential oil is unique in its ability to stop bacteria while promoting healthy skin. Because this treatment goes straight up your nose, be absolutely certain you are not sensitive to frankincense essential oil before use. Using a cotton swab, apply 1 or 2 drops of frankincense essential oil to the polyp. Repeat this treatment 2 times a day until the polyp has been eliminated.

TEA TREE TREATMENT

Tea tree essential oil stops bacterial activity while helping shrink and heal inflamed tissue. Because this treatment goes right up your nose, be absolutely certain you are not sensitive to tea tree essential oil before use. Using a cotton swab, apply 1 or 2 drops of tea tree essential oil to the polyp. Repeat this treatment 2 times a day until the polyp has been eliminated.

Natural Energy

Following a healthy diet, getting restful sleep, and maintaining an active lifestyle are some ways to keep your energy up. Use essential oils to complement a healthy lifestyle for an additional energy enhancement.

PEP UP WITH PEPPERMINT

Peppermint essential oil provides an almost instant feeling of rejuvenation, and may be used in a number of ways to increase energy naturally. Using your fingertip or a cotton swab, apply 1 drop of peppermint essential oil to each temple, or directly inhale the scent from the bottle. A few drops can also be added to a washcloth placed on the floor of your shower.

DIFFUSE LEMON AND GRAPEFRUIT

Lemon and grapefruit essential oils promote natural energy, increase alertness, and help your day move along. Diffuse a blend of equal amounts of lemon and grapefruit essential oils in the area where you spend the most time, or place the same blend inside an aromatherapy pendant. Incorporate 3 to 5 drops of the blend to add a delightful fragrance to natural shampoo, conditioner, and shower gel.

Nausea

Many illnesses are accompanied by nausea, which is the feeling of queasiness that warns you that vomiting may be imminent. Nausea is sometimes accompanied by a warm, uncomfortable feeling that spreads through your body; a feeling of dizziness or wooziness may also accompany it. If nausea happens frequently for no apparent reason, see your doctor, as an underlying medical condition could be present.

FENNEL COMPRESS

MAKES 1 TREATMENT

Fennel essential oil offers fast relief from nausea, particularly when applied with the aid of a hot compress. This remedy is not suitable for children, nor is it safe for women who are pregnant.

1 tablespoon carrier oil
4 drops fennel essential oil
1 pint hot water

1. In a small glass bowl, add the carrier oil and fennel essential oil, and stir to combine.
2. Using your fingertips, apply the blend to the upper abdomen.
3. In a medium bowl, add the hot water.
4. Submerge a towel in the water, wring it out, and apply the compress to the affected area. Leave the compress in place until it cools to body temperature.
5. Repeat this treatment every 2 to 3 hours as needed.

GINGER SMELLING SALTS

MAKES 1 TREATMENT

Ginger essential oil is among the best remedies available for nausea, and is suitable for anyone who is suffering from an upset stomach. Allspice (also known as pimento) essential oil intensifies the effect; however, it may be omitted if it is not available. This remedy can be used by children and women who are pregnant.

1 tablespoon sea salt
6 drops ginger essential oil
1 drop allspice (or pimento) essential oil

1. In a dark-colored glass bottle, add the sea salt along with the ginger and allspice essential oils, and shake well to blend.
2. Inhale from the bottle when feeling nauseous.
3. Repeat this treatment as needed.

Neck Pain

Neck pain is often mild, and is caused by muscle strain, poor posture, or other environmental issues; in some cases neck pain accompanies tension headaches. Essential oils can help relieve neck pain in these cases; if pain is severe, has been caused by trauma, or is ongoing with no evident cause, see your doctor for a diagnosis. Neck pain can be symptomatic of numerous severe diseases and should not be allowed to go undiagnosed.

PEPPERMINT PAIN RELIEF

Peppermint essential oil penetrates rapidly to relieve muscles while its vapors help the mind let go of worries that may be causing tension. For fast relief from neck pain, apply 10 drops of peppermint essential oil to the palm of one hand, then rub your hands together to distribute the oil. Massage the back of your neck with both hands, then sit or lie back comfortably with your back and neck aligned. Allow yourself to rest for at least 10 minutes before resuming normal activity.

CORIANDER MASSAGE

MAKES 1 TREATMENT

Coriander essential oil is an effective topical analgesic that also has the ability to relax the mind and promote feelings of well-being. It is also helpful for alleviating arthritic pain.

1 tablespoon carrier oil
8 drops coriander essential oil

1. In a small glass bowl, add the carrier oil and coriander essential oil, and stir to combine.
2. Using your fingertips, apply the blend to the back of the neck, and massage it into the skin.
3. Allow yourself to rest for at least 10 minutes before resuming normal activity.
4. Repeat this treatment up to 3 times a day until the pain subsides.

Nervousness

Whether from stage fright, anxiety about performing well at a new job, or for countless other reasons, nervousness is something that affects almost everyone at some time. Essential oils can help counteract the feelings of tension and near-panic that often accompany nervousness. If you are often nervous and no cause is apparent, see your doctor to rule out a serious disorder.

DIFFUSE CLARY SAGE

Clary sage essential oil dispels nervousness and anxiety rapidly, replacing them with feelings of well-being and contentment. Diffuse the essential oil in the area where you spend the most time, or carry it with you in an aromatherapy pendant. A few drops can be added to your bath or to a washcloth placed on the floor of your shower.

CLARY SAGE SMELLING SALTS

MAKES 1 TREATMENT

Clary sage essential oil is the perfect tool for getting rid of stage fright and other forms of nervousness that interrupt your daily life. Whether you are going for an important interview or partaking in a social situation where awkwardness threatens to intervene, these smelling salts prove helpful.

1 tablespoon sea salt
16 drops clary sage essential oil

1. In a dark-colored glass bottle, add the sea salt and clary sage essential oil, and shake well to blend.
2. Inhale from the bottle.
3. Repeat this treatment as needed.

Norovirus

Also known as Norwalk virus, norovirus is typically spread via contaminated food and water, though it can be passed from person to person. Gastrointestinal distress, vomiting, diarrhea, headache, and a low fever of less than 100 degrees Fahrenheit are typically present. Essential oils provide comfort and alleviate symptoms in most cases; few symptoms become severe or require medical attention.

MELISSA BATH OIL

MAKES 1 TREATMENT

Melissa essential oil has both antispasmodic and stomachic properties. These, along with its other properties, make melissa essential oil ideal for alleviating the gastrointestinal problems that accompany norovirus. Melissa essential oil also eases headache and fever, making it a top pick for this and similar illnesses.

1 tablespoon carrier oil
8 drops melissa essential oil

1. In a small glass bowl, add the carrier oil and melissa essential oil, and stir to combine.
2. Draw a warm bath and add the entire treatment to the running water.
3. Soak for at least 15 minutes. Use caution when getting out of the bathtub, as it may be slippery.
4. Repeat this treatment up to 3 times a day until symptoms subside.

PALMAROSA COMPRESS

MAKES 1 TREATMENT

Palmarosa essential oil helps alleviate fever, clear intestinal infections, and aid the digestive system. Its fragrance is uplifting, helping eliminate the exhaustion that accompanies illness.

1 teaspoon carrier oil
4 drops palmarosa essential oil
1 pint cold water

1. Using your fingertips, apply the carrier oil to the abdomen, followed by the palmarosa essential oil.
2. In a medium glass bowl, add the cold water.
3. Submerge a towel in the water, wring it out, and apply the compress to the affected area. Leave the compress in place until it warms to body temperature.
4. Reapply the compress until the water has lost its chill.
5. Repeat this treatment up to 3 times a day until symptoms subside.

Nosebleed

Although nosebleeds are not typically serious, they can be alarming. Often triggered by trauma or prolonged exposure to dry indoor air, nosebleeds are easy to treat. If nosebleeds are frequent, are accompanied by other symptoms, or are the result of a severe trauma, see a doctor.

ROSE GERANIUM NASAL POULTICE

MAKES 1 TREATMENT

Rose geranium essential oil is a styptic substance, meaning it can help staunch the flow of blood. It also helps promote tissue healing, making it ideal for stopping and treating bloody noses.

10 drops rose geranium essential oil
1 small tampon

1. Drip the rose geranium essential oil on the end of the tampon, then insert it into the affected nostril.
2. Leave the tampon in place for at least 10 minutes before carefully removing it.

LEMON-LAVENDER INHALATION

MAKES 1 TREATMENT

Lavender and lemon essential oils soothe the feelings of alarm that often accompany nosebleeds while helping stop bacterial activity. Because this treatment involves pinching the nostrils closed, use it only if your nosebleed was not caused by trauma to the nose.

2 drops lemon essential oil
1 drop lavender essential oil

1. Drip the lemon and lavender essential oils on a tissue, then inhale deeply, taking between 10 and 15 breaths in through your nose and out your mouth.
2. Put the tissue aside and pinch your nostrils closed for 10 minutes.
3. If desired, place an ice pack on the bridge of your nose to help stop the bleeding.

Oil Pulling

Oil pulling is a traditional Ayurveda practice. Essential oils, in combination with edible oils, are swished and held in the mouth to promote oral health, prevent bad breath, heal gums, and detoxify the body. Major studies have shown that oil pulling can kill the bacteria that cause cavities, making it a good alternative to brushing with fluoride toothpaste.

GRAPEFRUIT DETOX

MAKES 1 TREATMENT

Grapefruit essential oil is an excellent detoxifier, with antibacterial and antiseptic qualities that help promote dental and general health.

1 tablespoon coconut or sunflower carrier oil
2 drops grapefruit essential oil

1. In a small glass bowl, add the coconut carrier oil and grapefruit essential oil, and stir to combine.
2. Swish the mixture in your mouth and suck it through your teeth slowly. Try to make the treatment last for 15 minutes. If you are new to oil pulling, start with a few minutes and increase the amount of the treatment over time.
3. Spit the oil out when finished, then brush your teeth and rinse your mouth with water.
4. Repeat this treatment once a day upon waking.

TEA TREE COLD AND FLU TREATMENT

MAKES 1 TREATMENT

Tea tree essential oil is ideal for oil pulling when cold or flu symptoms start to rear their heads. You can also use it as a general dental cleanser that helps put a stop to gingivitis and other oral complications.

1 tablespoon coconut or sunflower carrier oil
2 drops tea tree essential oil

1. In a small glass bowl, add the coconut carrier oil and tea tree essential oil, and stir to combine.
2. Swish the mixture through your mouth and suck it through your teeth slowly. Try to make the treatment last for 15 minutes. If you are new to oil pulling, start with a few minutes and increase the amount of the treatment over time.
3. Spit the oil out when finished, then brush your teeth and rinse your mouth with water.
4. Repeat this treatment once a day upon waking.

Oily Scalp

Itchiness, flaky skin, and a general feeling of discomfort often accompany an overly oily scalp. In some cases, bacteria begin to feed on excess scalp oil, leading to an unpleasant odor. Use essential oils to alleviate the unsightly appearance of excessive oiliness.

CEDARWOOD SCALP TONIC

MAKES 24 TREATMENTS

Cedarwood essential oil helps balance sebum production. In addition, it is antibacterial and leaves a delightful fragrance behind.

4 ounces water

24 drops cedarwood essential oil

1. In a dark-colored glass bottle fitted with a spray top, add the water and cedarwood essential oil, and shake well to blend.
2. Spray the scalp generously, either after shampooing and conditioning, or at any other time.
3. Massage the blend in, then comb the hair and style as usual.
4. Repeat this treatment up to 2 times per day. Shake the bottle before each use.

GRAPEFRUIT-LEMON SCALP TONIC

MAKES 1 TREATMENT

Grapefruit and lemon essential oils are astringents; they help stop excess oil production and leave the hair looking shiny and clean.

1 tablespoon warm water

4 drops grapefruit essential oil

3 drops lemon essential oil

1. In a small glass bowl, add the warm water along with the grapefruit and lemon essential oils, and stir to combine.
2. Using your fingertips, apply the entire blend to the scalp after shampooing and conditioning the hair.
3. Massage the blend in, then comb the hair and style as usual.
4. Repeat this treatment once a day.

Oily Skin

The skin produces oil to protect itself from outside elements that cause dryness. When too much oil is produced, the skin looks shiny and feels uncomfortably heavy. Although oily skin is primarily a cosmetic complaint, complications such as acne can occur.

FENNEL FACIAL TONER

MAKES 24 TREATMENTS

Fennel is an excellent addition to facial toner, as its antiseptic properties make it useful in stopping minor infections that often accompany excessively oily skin.

1 ounce witch hazel
8 drops fennel essential oil

1. In a dark-colored glass bottle, add the witch hazel and fennel essential oil, and shake well to blend.
2. Using a cotton pad, apply a few drops to the face and other oily areas.
3. Repeat this treatment up to 2 times a day. Shake the bottle before each use.

BALANCING CITRUS TONER

MAKES 24 TREATMENTS

Grapefruit and lemon essential oils are strong astringents that can help balance the skin and eliminate excessive oil. If this recipe is overly drying for your skin, replace the vodka with witch hazel or water. Do not use this treatment with children.

1 ounce vodka
7 drops grapefruit essential oil
5 drops lemon essential oil

1. In a dark-colored glass bottle, add the vodka along with the grapefruit and lemon essential oils, and shake well to blend.
2. Using a cotton pad, apply a few drops to the face and other oily areas.
3. Repeat this treatment up to 2 times a day. Shake the bottle before each use.

Pain Management

Many conditions cause pain; some are minor, and some are both chronic and severe. Essential oils can be used as part of a pain management plan. See your doctor if you have serious or chronic undiagnosed pain, as it may be symptomatic of an underlying medical condition.

CINNAMON BATH OIL

MAKES 8 TREATMENTS

Cinnamon essential oil is a strong analgesic. Its heat penetrates deep into tissue, promoting relaxation and helping ease even the worst chronic pain. Check for sensitivity to the essential oil before use. Those who are pregnant or who have cancer should not use this treatment.

4 ounces carrier oil
20 drops cinnamon essential oil

1. In a dark-colored glass bottle, add the carrier oil and cinnamon essential oil, and shake well to blend.
2. Draw a warm bath and add 1 tablespoon of the blend to the running water.
3. Soak for at least 15 minutes. Use caution when getting out of the bathtub, as it may be slippery.
4. Repeat this treatment up to 2 times a day as needed.

EUCALYPTUS COMPRESS

MAKES 1 TREATMENT

Eucalyptus essential oil is an effective analgesic that also helps tight tissue to relax. A hot compress intensifies its effects.

1 teaspoon carrier oil
8 drops eucalyptus essential oil
1 pint hot water

1. Using your fingertip, apply the carrier oil to the affected area, followed by the eucalyptus essential oil.
2. In a medium glass bowl, add the hot water.
3. Submerge a towel in the water, wring it out, and apply the compress to the affected area. Layer plastic wrap on top of the compress to keep the essential oil vapors from evaporating. Leave the compress in place until it cools to body temperature.
4. Repeat this treatment every 2 to 3 hours until symptoms subside.

Parkinson's Disease

Parkinson's disease is a neurodegenerative disorder characterized by a progressive inability to control the muscles, leading to trembling, slowness, stiffness, and impaired balance. As the disease progresses, moving, talking, and completing even simple tasks become more difficult. Use essential oils to complement conventional therapy with your caregiver's approval.

SUBLINGUAL FRANKINCENSE

Frankincense essential oil has a positive effect on the mind and body, calming the mind, promoting relaxed, even breathing, and stopping anxiety. It also aids in promoting muscle function, particularly with respect to small, smooth muscles. Take 1 drop of frankincense essential oil sublingually each day as a tonic to support overall well-being.

DIFFUSE FRANKINCENSE AND MYRRH

Frankincense and myrrh promote mental balance and decrease the anxiety and agitation that often accompanies Parkinson's disease. The fragrance is warm, spicy, and comforting. Diffuse equal amounts of frankincense and myrrh in the area where the patient spends most of his time.

Periodontal Disease

Periodontal disease is a severe form of gum disease that typically begins with gingivitis. Use essential oils to restore health in minor cases of periodontal disease. If the disease is advanced, seek medical intervention.

MYRRH MOUTHWASH

MAKES 1 TREATMENT

Myrrh is a potent antibacterial, and is ideal for flushing the gums and teeth of plaque and food particles that can complicate periodontal disease.

1 tablespoon water
4 drops myrrh essential oil

1. In a small glass bowl, add the water and myrrh essential oil, and stir to combine.
2. Swish the blend through entire mouth, pulling it through the teeth with gentle suction. Try to make the treatment last for 10 minutes.
3. Spit the oil out when finished, then brush your teeth and rinse your mouth.
4. Repeat this treatment at least once a day.

LAVENDER GUM TONIC

MAKES 1 TREATMENT

Lavender soothes pain, kills bacteria, and promotes healing. This remedy does not taste nice; however, it is effective in healing sore, compromised gums. Use this treatment after brushing your teeth.

1 tablespoon water
8 drops lavender essential oil

1. In a small glass bowl, add the water and lavender essential oil, and stir to combine.
2. Swish the blend through the entire mouth, pulling it through the teeth with gentle suction. Try to make it last for 5 minutes.
3. Spit the oil out when finished. Do not eat or drink anything for 30 minutes afterward.
4. Repeat this treatment once a day until the gum condition improves.

Plantar Fasciitis

Plantar fasciitis is foot and heel pain caused when the plantar fascia, which is the ligament connecting the toes to the heel bone and supporting the arch of the foot, undergoes repeated strain. Swelling, weakness, and inflammation may be present. Essential oils should be used in conjunction with appropriate footwear, rest, and elevation. The worst cases call for surgical intervention. See your doctor if treatment at home does not bring relief.

NUMB PAIN WITH CLOVE

Clove essential oil is a powerful numbing agent that eases pain and helps the tiny muscles in your foot relax. Apply a few drops of clove essential oil to the area where pain is worst, then prop your feet up and rest for a while. Repeat this treatment once a day as needed.

HELICHRYSUM-PEPPERMINT COMPRESS

MAKES 1 TREATMENT

Helichrysum and peppermint come together to alleviate pain and aid in healing; a warm compress helps keep the vapors contained.

12 drops helichrysum essential oil
3 drops peppermint essential oil
1 teaspoon carrier oil
1 pint hot water

1. Using your fingertips, apply the helichrysum essential oil to where the pain is worst, followed by the peppermint essential oil, then the carrier oil.
2. In a medium glass bowl, pour the hot water.
3. Submerge a towel in the water, wring it out, and apply the compress to the affected area. Layer plastic wrap on top of the compress to keep the essential oil vapors from evaporating. Leave the compress in place until it cools to body temperature.
4. Repeat this treatment 2 times a day—when waking, before putting on socks and shoes, and at bedtime—until symptoms subside.

Pneumonia

Pneumonia often follows on the heels of a cold, the flu, or an upper-respiratory infection. Symptoms include a cough with green or blood-tinged mucus, chills and shaking, pain in the chest wall that worsens with breathing or coughing, and feelings of weakness and tiredness. Healthy people often have mild symptoms that don't require medical intervention; however, babies, children, elderly people, and anyone with compromised health should see a doctor, as pneumonia can worsen rapidly.

CYPRESS BATH

MAKES 1 TREATMENT

Cypress essential oil has strong warming properties, making it a great essential oil to combat the chills of pneumonia.

1 tablespoon carrier oil
5 drops cypress essential oil

1. In a small glass bowl, add the carrier oil and cypress essential oil, and stir to combine.
2. Draw a warm bath and add the entire treatment to the running water.
3. Soak for at least 15 minutes. Use caution when getting out of the bathtub, as it may be slippery.
4. Repeat this treatment up to 5 times a day as needed.

NIAOULI BATH

MAKES 1 TREATMENT

Niaouli essential oil is an effective antiseptic and an excellent remedy for easing pneumonia symptoms. This bath allows you to benefit by absorption and by breathing the vapors.

1 tablespoon carrier oil
8 drops niaouli essential oil

1. In a small glass bowl, add the carrier oil and niaouli essential oil, and stir to combine.
2. Draw a warm bath and add the entire treatment to the running water.
3. Soak for at least 15 minutes. Use caution when getting out of the bathtub, as it may be slippery.
4. Repeat this treatment up to 4 times a day as needed.

Poison Ivy

With exposure to poison ivy, poison oak, or poison sumac come redness, swelling, and unbearable itching; burning pain is sometimes present, too, as are blisters. While essential oils help in the majority of cases, some of the most severe reactions require medical attention. If the eyes or mucus membranes are involved, or if you have been exposed to smoke caused by burning poison ivy or related plants, seek emergency treatment immediately.

FRANKINCENSE-PEPPERMINT SPRAY

MAKES 24 TREATMENTS

Frankincense and peppermint essential oils combine to take the heat, itching, and pain out of poison ivy while promoting healing. Apply this remedy only after you have completely cleansed the area.

1 ounce water
20 drops frankincense essential oil
20 drops peppermint essential oil

1. In a dark-colored glass bottle fitted with a spray top, add the water along with the frankincense and peppermint essential oils, and shake well to blend.
2. Spray the affected area generously, allowing it to dry before dressing.
3. Repeat this treatment as needed. Shake the bottle before each use.

LAVENDER-MYRRH SALVE

MAKES 10 TREATMENTS

Lavender and myrrh essential oils numb the pain poison ivy causes while helping the skin heal faster. If the area is too painful to touch, put the salve in a small spray bottle and mist it on.

1 teaspoon carrier oil
20 drops lavender essential oil
10 drops myrrh essential oil

1. In a dark-colored glass bottle, add the carrier oil along with the lavender and myrrh essential oils, and shake well to blend.
2. Using a cotton pad, apply the blend to the affected area, dabbing rather than wiping.
3. Repeat the treatment as needed. Shake the bottle before each use.

Postpartum

During the six weeks following childbirth, your body is healing and adjusting to not being pregnant. Soreness, afterpains, and a small amount of bleeding may occur, along with extreme tiredness. If you begin to feel depressed or feel like hurting yourself or your baby, seek treatment. Postpartum depression requires immediate intervention.

JASMINE-ROSE BATH

MAKES 1 TREATMENT

Jasmine and rose essential oils support mental balance, help ease emotional stress, and soothe frayed nerves while promoting glowing skin and helping taxed tissues to heal.

1 tablespoon carrier oil
10 drops jasmine essential oil
10 drops rose essential oil

1. In a small glass bowl, add the carrier oil along with the jasmine and rose essential oils, and stir to combine.
2. Draw a warm bath and add the entire treatment to the running water.
3. Soak for at least 15 minutes. Use caution when getting out of the bathtub, as it may be slippery.
4. Repeat this treatment 1 or 2 times a day for 2 to 6 weeks after birth.

PERINEUM CARE SPRAY

MAKES 24 TREATMENTS

Frankincense, helichrysum, and lavender essential oils help sore or compromised perineum tissue heal faster while providing pain relief naturally.

4 ounces water
24 drops frankincense essential oil
24 drops helichrysum essential oil
24 drops lavender essential oil

1. In a dark-colored glass bottle fitted with a spray top, add the water along with the frankincense, helichrysum, and lavender essential oils, and shake well to blend.
2. Spray the affected area generously.
3. Repeat this treatment as needed until healed. Shake the bottle before each use.

Premenstrual Syndrome (PMS)

Premenstrual syndrome (PMS) is characterized by symptoms that include mood swings, sadness, irritability, bloating, indigestion, cramps, carb cravings, sleep problems, headache, and breast tenderness. Symptoms range in severity, and the effectiveness of treatment with essential oils varies from one woman to the next. If pain and other symptoms are severe, see your doctor for an evaluation, as these could be indicative of an underlying condition.

IMPROVE MOOD WITH CLARY SAGE

Clary sage essential oil is known to uplift the mood. This treatment can be applied in several ways. Diffuse clary sage essential oil in the area where you spend the most time, place it in an aromatherapy pendant, or add 2 or 3 drops to your bath or to a washcloth placed on the floor of your shower. Repeat this treatment as needed to keep your mood stable.

LEMONGRASS BATH

MAKES 1 TREATMENT

Lemongrass essential oil helps stop bloating associated with PMS; at the same time, it helps stop muscle pain associated with cramping. As an added benefit, it revitalizes the mind and helps alleviate stress.

1 tablespoon carrier oil
8 drops lemongrass essential oil

1. In a small glass bowl, add the carrier oil and lemongrass essential oil, and stir to combine.
2. Draw a warm bath and add the entire treatment to the running water.
3. Soak for at least 15 minutes. Use caution when getting out of the bathtub, as it may be slippery.
4. Repeat this treatment once a day as needed.

CLARY SAGE BATH

MAKES 1 TREATMENT

Clary sage essential oil is among the most effective womb tonics available; it helps ease painful periods while addressing emotional turmoil and promoting feelings of calm and overall well-being. If you suspect tender breasts, irritability, and weight gain could be due to pregnancy, do not use this remedy, as clary sage stimulates menstruation.

1 tablespoon carrier oil
10 drops clary sage essential oil

1. In a small glass bowl, add the carrier oil and clary sage essential oil, and stir to combine.
2. Draw a warm bath and add the entire treatment to the running water.
3. Soak for at least 15 minutes. Use caution when getting out of the bathtub, as it may be slippery.
4. Repeat this treatment once a day as needed.

FRANKINCENSE-MELISSA SOAK

MAKES 1 TREATMENT

Frankincense essential oil is an effective womb tonic that helps ease heavy periods while melissa essential oil has antispasmodic properties that help put a stop to cramps. This treatment has a lovely fragrance that soothes nervous tension and alleviates crankiness; as melissa essential oil is a fairly potent sedative, it is best to use this treatment in the evening.

1 tablespoon carrier oil
8 drops frankincense essential oil
8 drops melissa essential oil

1. In a small glass bowl, add the carrier oil along with the frankincense and melissa essential oils, and stir to combine.
2. Draw a warm bath and add the entire treatment to the running water.
3. Soak for at least 15 minutes. Use caution when getting out of the bathtub, as it may be slippery.
4. Repeat this treatment once a day as needed.

Prostatitis

Sometimes described simply as an infection of the prostate gland, prostatitis is often nothing more than inflammation. It can affect men of all ages, and it is sometimes related to urinary tract infections. Frequent urination, an urgent need to urinate, and general pain throughout the pelvic area are symptoms of prostatitis. If more severe symptoms such as burning pain, fever, chills, or nausea and vomiting are present, seek medical attention. Left untreated, severe cases of prostatitis can prove fatal.

JUNIPER-BERGAMOT BATH

MAKES 1 TREATMENT

Juniper, lavender, and bergamot essential oils help stop the discomfort of prostatitis and soothe inflammation.

1 tablespoon carrier oil
6 drops juniper essential oil
4 drops lavender essential oil
2 drops bergamot essential oil

1. In a small glass bowl, add the carrier oil along with the juniper, lavender, and bergamot essential oils, and stir to combine.
2. Draw a warm bath and add the entire treatment to the running water.
3. Soak for at least 15 minutes. Use caution when getting out of the bathtub, as it may be slippery.
4. Repeat this treatment up to 3 times a day.

HEALING PINE MASSAGE OIL

MAKES 1 TREATMENT

Pine essential oil has an intense warming quality and is an effective antiseptic. Do not allow this remedy to come into contact with sensitive membranes.

1 teaspoon carrier oil
6 drops pine essential oil

1. In a small glass bowl, add the carrier oil and pine essential oil, and stir to combine.
2. Using your fingertips, apply the blend to the external prostate area, and massage it into the skin. Applying the blend to the lower back may also be helpful.
3. Repeat this treatment up to 3 times a day.

Psoriasis

Psoriasis is typically characterized by bright red, raised patches of skin covered with loose white to silver scales, normally on the elbows, knees, or back. Bleeding, crusting, and severe itching are common, and in some cases, pitted or discolored nails occur. Seek medical intervention as soon as you notice signs of psoriasis, as early treatment can prevent the problem from becoming worse. In addition, seek treatment if you notice red streaks, more pain, swelling, or redness than normal, or the formation of pus. Use essential oil as a complementary therapy with your doctor's approval.

NEAT CARROT SEED TREATMENT

Carrot seed essential oil detoxifies the skin, adds elasticity, and stimulates healthy regrowth of damaged tissue. At the same time, it soothes the pain psoriasis brings with it. Apply a small amount of carrot seed essential oil to the affected areas, either using your fingertips or a cotton pad. Repeat this treatment at least 2 times a day to promote healing.

JUNIPER BATH

MAKES 1 TREATMENT

Juniper essential oil is a strong antiseptic and astringent, which helps ease the pain and discomfort of psoriasis while promoting healing.

1 tablespoon carrier oil
7 drops juniper essential oil

1. In a small glass bowl, add the carrier oil and juniper essential oil, and stir to combine.
2. Draw a warm bath and add the entire treatment to the running water.
3. Soak for at least 15 minutes. Use caution when getting out of the bathtub, as it may be slippery.
4. Repeat this treatment up to 3 times a day until symptoms subside.

Radiation Therapy

Radiation therapy can cause a number of side effects, ranging from nausea and fatigue to hair loss and skin problems. Essential oils are not meant to replace radiation therapy; instead, they are tools you can use to bring comfort and reduce the stress that can make side effects worse.

DIFFUSE FRANKINCENSE

Frankincense essential oil has a strongly positive effect on the mind, helping alleviate anxiety and ward off depression. It can help you stop focusing on fear and pay more attention to the good things in life. Diffuse frankincense essential oil in the area where you spend the most time, and consider carrying it with you in an aromatherapy pendant. You can also add 2 or 3 drops to your bath, where, as an added benefit, the essential oil helps keep compromised skin supple.

MOISTURIZING ROSE-GERANIUM OIL

MAKES 8 TREATMENTS

Geranium and rose essential oils nourish skin and promote increased elasticity while their fragrances soothe and uplift the mind. This treatment will not stop radiation or chemo-therapy from changing your skin, but it can help you deal with the changes that occur.

4 ounces carrier oil
16 drops geranium essential oil
16 drops rose essential oil

1. In a dark-colored glass bottle, add the carrier oil along with the geranium and rose essential oils, and shake well to blend.
2. Using your fingertips, apply 1 tablespoon to the body after bathing or showering, and massage it into the skin.
3. Repeat this treatment once a day as needed.

Razor Bumps

Razor bumps develop after shaving, when hair curls back on itself and grows into the skin rather than growing up and away from the skin. These small bumps are often irritated, can contain pus, and can lead to scarring. If your razor bumps do not respond to treatment with essential oils and become worse, you may need to stop shaving or choose a different method of hair removal.

NEAT TEA TREE TREATMENT

Tea tree essential oil stops infection and helps shrink inflamed tissue so razor bumps don't look or feel quite so bad. Apply a few drops of tea tree essential oil to the affected area after cleansing your skin but before moisturizing. Allow the essential oil to dry completely before moisturizing or putting on your clothes. Repeat this treatment once a day.

SOOTHING LAVENDER SPRAY

MAKES 24 TREATMENTS

Lavender essential oil helps shrink inflamed tissue while stopping infection and alleviating discomfort. This simple spray leaves a lovely fragrance behind.

4 ounces water
48 drops lavender essential oil

1. In a dark-colored glass bottle fitted with a spray top, add the water and lavender essential oil, and shake well to blend.
2. Spray the blend on the affected area.
3. Repeat this treatment as needed to stop itching. Shake the bottle before each use.

Restless Legs Syndrome

Restless legs syndrome (RLS) is accompanied by a strong urge to move while attempting to fall asleep. Uncomfortable or painful sensations are common, and though they normally affect the legs, they may affect any part of the body. RLS symptoms tend to begin about 15 minutes after relaxing, and periodic limb movements may occur after you fall asleep. Essential oils combined with regular exercise may be enough in minor cases. See your doctor if these treatments do not work, as RLS can sometimes be symptomatic of an underlying medical condition such as anemia or diabetes.

CHAMOMILE SALVE

MAKES 1 TREATMENT

Chamomile promotes relaxation and helps ease the worry and mental turmoil that often accompanies restless legs syndrome.

1 tablespoon carrier oil
12 drops Roman chamomile essential oil

1. In a small glass bowl, add the carrier oil and Roman chamomile essential oil, and stir to combine.
2. Using your fingertips, apply the blend to the legs, and massage it vigorously into the skin.
3. Repeat this treatment as needed.

LAVENDER-FRANKINCENSE MASSAGE

MAKES 1 TREATMENT

Frankincense and lavender essential oils promote general well-being, ease tension, and help stop mental anguish.

1 tablespoon carrier oil
10 drops lavender essential oil
5 drops frankincense essential oil

1. In a small glass bowl, add the carrier oil along with the lavender and frankincense essential oils, and stir to combine.
2. Using your fingertips, apply the blend to the legs, and massage it vigorously into the skin.
3. Repeat this treatment once a day before bedtime, and focus on the fragrance as you fall asleep.

Rheumatoid Arthritis

Rheumatoid arthritis is accompanied by symptoms that include joint stiffness, painful joints, fever, and fatigue. Essential oils can bring comfort and replace some pain medications, particularly in mild cases. See your doctor if home treatment is not helping or symptoms are becoming worse.

JUNIPER COMPRESS

MAKES 1 TREATMENT

Juniper essential oil is an effective antirheumatic, which helps alleviate the pain of swollen joints and sore muscles.

8 drops juniper essential oil
1 teaspoon carrier oil
1 pint hot water

1. Using your fingertips, apply the juniper essential oil to sore muscles, followed by the carrier oil.
2. In a medium glass bowl, add the hot water.
3. Submerge a towel in the water, wring it out, and apply the compress to the affected area. Layer plastic wrap on top of the compress to keep the essential oil vapors from evaporating. Leave the compress in place until it warms to body temperature.
4. Repeat this treatment up to 3 times a day as needed.

VETIVER AND YLANG-YLANG BATH

MAKES 1 TREATMENT

Vetiver essential oil is a potent antirheumatic, easing pain, soothing the mind, and dispelling worry. Ylang-ylang essential oil promotes feelings of overall well-being while giving this bath a lovely fragrance.

1 tablespoon carrier oil
6 drops vetiver essential oil
6 drops ylang-ylang essential oil

1. In a small glass bowl, add the carrier oil along with the vetiver and ylang-ylang essential oils, and stir to combine.
2. Draw a warm bath and add the entire treatment to the running water.
3. Soak for at least 15 minutes. Use caution when getting out of the bathtub, as it may be slippery.
4. Repeat this treatment once a day as needed.

Ringworm

Ringworm is a fungal infection of the skin. Characterized by circular red patches with raised borders, severe itching, and a tendency to spread rapidly, ringworm is highly contagious but responds very well to treatment. If your rash develops blisters or appears to be infected, seek medical treatment; antibiotics are often prescribed when home treatments fail.

NEAT TEA TREE TREATMENT

Tea tree essential oil soothes the itching and pain that accompany ringworm and effectively kills the fungus that causes it. Using a cotton swab, apply a small amount of tea tree essential oil to each affected area. Repeat this treatment 2 times a day until the ringworm fades.

TRIPLE-OIL RINGWORM TREATMENT

MAKES 10 TREATMENTS

A more fragrant and somewhat milder approach than applying tea tree oil neat, this remedy incorporates lavender essential oil to soothe inflammation and stop itching, plus tea tree and thyme essential oils to kill the fungus.

30 drops carrier oil
30 drops lavender essential oil
30 drops tea tree essential oil
30 drops thyme essential oil

1. In a dark-colored glass bottle, add the carrier oil along with the lavender, tea tree, and thyme essential oils, and shake well to mix.
2. Using a cotton swab, apply a small amount of the blend to each affected area.
3. Repeat this treatment 2 times a day until the ringworm fades.

Rocky Mountain Spotted Fever

Rocky Mountain spotted fever (RMSF) is an infectious disease transmitted by ticks. Symptoms include severe headaches, a high fever, muscle pain, abdominal pain, and loss of appetite along with a distinctive rash with small, flat reddish spots. Despite its name, RMSF has been reported throughout the United States as well as Canada, Mexico, South America, and Central America. See your doctor if you suspect a case of RMSF, as life-threatening complications can occur. Use essential oils to provide comfort in conjunction with medical treatment.

FENNEL-SANDALWOOD BATH

MAKES 1 TREATMENT

Fennel essential oil helps promote skin healing while addressing pain and discomfort. Sandalwood essential oil is a strong antiseptic that helps relieve symptoms.

1 tablespoon carrier oil
4 drops fennel essential oil
2 drops sandalwood essential oil

1. In a small glass bowl, add the carrier oil along with the fennel and sandalwood essential oils, and stir to combine.
2. Draw a warm bath and add the entire treatment to the running water.
3. Soak for at least 15 minutes. Use caution when getting out of the bathtub, as it may be slippery.
4. Repeat this treatment once a day as needed.

GINGER-BERGAMOT BATH

MAKES 1 TREATMENT

Ginger essential oil helps stop pain and treat gastric distress. In addition, it may help you regain your appetite. The bergamot essential oil helps reduce fevers and ease discomfort.

1 tablespoon carrier oil
3 drops ginger essential oil
2 drops bergamot essential oil

1. In a small glass bowl, add the carrier oil along with the ginger and bergamot essential oils, and stir to combine.
2. Draw a warm bath and add the entire treatment to the running water.
3. Soak for at least 15 minutes. Use caution when getting out of the bathtub, as it may be slippery.
4. Repeat this treatment once a day as needed.

Rosacea

Rosacea is sometimes referred to as adult acne due to the pimples that often accompany it. Rosacea may cause soreness and burning in the eye area, and it can sometimes lead to coarse, thickened facial skin. Essential oils can help alleviate rosacea symptoms, particularly when used in concert with other therapies such as laser and light treatment.

NEAT GERANIUM TREATMENT

Geranium essential oil soothes and heals troubled skin and is particularly helpful in softening thickened skin. Apply a small amount to your face after washing but before moisturizing. Repeat this treatment once a day to help alleviate symptoms. You may use rose geranium essential oil if you do not have geranium essential oil.

FRANKINCENSE-HELICHRYSUM BALM

MAKES 1 TREATMENT

Helichrysum essential oil helps soothe and heal compromised skin, and frankincense essential oil kills bacteria and aids in healing.

3 drops frankincense essential oil
3 drops helichrysum essential oil

1. In a small glass bowl, add the frankincense and helichrysum essential oils, and stir to combine.
2. Using your fingertips, apply the blend to the affected areas.
3. Repeat this treatment at least once a day after washing your face and before moisturizing.

Runny Nose

A runny nose is often symptomatic of another problem such as a cold, flu, or allergies.

TEA TREE T-SHIRT TENT

MAKES 1 TREATMENT

This simple remedy eases the inflammation that causes excess mucus to release.

1 teaspoon carrier oil
4 drops tea tree essential oil

1. Using your fingertips, apply the carrier oil on your chest, followed by the tea tree essential oil.
2. Put on a clean crewneck T-shirt you don't mind staining with oil.
3. Sit comfortably and pull the neck of the T-shirt up over your nose and mouth, breathing deeply. Emerge for air when needed.
4. Keep breathing the essential oil until symptoms subside.
5. Repeat this treatment as needed.

LAVENDER-LEMON SMELLING SALTS

MAKES 1 TREATMENT

Both lavender and lemon essential oils help soothe inflamed sinuses and nasal passages.

1 tablespoon sea salt
10 drops lavender essential oil
4 drops lemon essential oil

1. In a dark-colored glass bottle, add the sea salt along with the lavender and lemon essential oils, and shake well to blend.
2. Inhale the blend.
3. Repeat this treatment as needed

Scabies

Scabies is caused by tiny mites that burrow into the skin, causing extreme itchiness. Left untreated, open sores and infection can develop. Because scabies is extremely contagious, all members of the family should be treated as soon as an infestation is discovered. The itching typically continues for two to four weeks after treatment has concluded. If symptoms recur or worsen, contact your doctor, as you may need a stronger treatment to eradicate the mites.

PEPPERMINT SALVE

MAKES 1 TREATMENT

Peppermint essential oil kills scabies while relieving the itching and burning that accompanies the parasites. This treatment may be too harsh for those with sensitive skin, in which case the tea tree essential oil remedy should be used instead.

1 teaspoon carrier oil
20 drops peppermint essential oil

1. In a small glass bowl, add the carrier oil and peppermint essential oil, and stir to combine.
2. Using your fingertips, apply the blend to the affected area.
3. Repeat this treatment 1 to 3 times a day for 3 days.

TEA TREE-LAVENDER SPRITZ

MAKES 16 TREATMENTS

Tea tree essential oil typically kills scabies within two to three days, and lavender essential oil helps promote healing.

1 teaspoon tea tree essential oil
1 teaspoon lavender essential oil

1. In a dark-colored glass bottle fitted with a spray top, add the lavender and tea tree essential oils, and shake well to blend.
2. Spray the blend onto the affected area.
3. Repeat this treatment 2 or 3 times a day for 2 to 3 days.

Scalp Psoriasis

Scalp psoriasis produces raised patches of scaly, reddish skin that sometimes affects only the scalp, forehead, behind the ears, and the back of the neck. Usually mild to moderate, scalp psoriasis tends to respond well to treatment with essential oils. In severe cases with crusted lesions and infection, you may need to see your doctor for a stronger remedy.

CARROT SEED HOT OIL TREATMENT

MAKES 1 TREATMENT

Carrot seed essential oil promotes healing, rejuvenating and stimulating skin while fighting psoriasis and other painful, itchy conditions.

1 tablespoon carrier oil
10 drops carrot seed essential oil

1. In a dark-colored glass bottle, add the carrier oil and carrot seed essential oil, and shake well to blend.
2. Set the bottle in a larger container filled with 1 inch of hot water and leave it there for 5 minutes to warm the oil.
3. Pour the entire blend over damp hair, and massage it gently into the skin.
4. Leave the treatment in place for at least 30 minutes, then shampoo, condition, and style your hair as usual.
5. Repeat this treatment up to 3 times a day until symptoms subside.

JUNIPER SCALP SPRITZ

MAKES 24 TREATMENTS

Juniper essential oil helps stop the pain and itching associated with scalp psoriasis while promoting healing.

4 ounces water
24 drops juniper essential oil

1. In a dark-colored glass bottle fitted with a spray top, add the water and juniper essential oil, and shake well to blend.
2. Spray the blend on the affected area after washing the hair. Allow the hair to dry and style as usual.
3. Repeat this treatment 2 times a day until symptoms subside.

Scarring

Scars develop when the skin heals after trauma. You can reduce scarring by taking good care of wounds when they occur, and some scars can be effectively diminished by treatment with essential oils.

NEAT HELICHRYSUM TREATMENT

Helichrysum essential oil is an extremely effective skin tonic, promoting tissue regeneration, softening, and diminishing the likelihood that heavy scarring will occur after an injury. Apply just enough helichrysum essential oil to cover the scrape or cut as it heals to help prevent scars. Repeat the treatment up to 3 times a day until the wound heals.

HYSSOP SALVE

MAKES 12 TREATMENTS

Hyssop essential oil is an antiseptic that stimulates healthy skin regeneration and stops inflammation. When used diligently following an injury, it can prevent serious scarring.

2 tablespoons carrier oil
24 drops hyssop essential oil

1. In a dark-colored glass bottle, add the carrier oil and hyssop essential oil.
2. Using your fingertips, apply approximately ½ teaspoon of the blend to the affected area. Allow the skin to dry before dressing.
3. Repeat this treatment 2 or 3 times a day until the wound heals.

Sciatica

Sciatica occurs when the sciatic nerve, which begins in the lower back and runs through the back side of the legs, is compromised for some reason. Symptoms include shooting pains, leg weakness, pain in the legs when sitting, and low back pain. If essential oils and stretching don't help ease the pain, see your doctor; sciatica can be symptomatic of degenerative disc disease and other serious conditions.

BERGAMOT TREATMENT

Bergamot essential oil is a strong anti-inflammatory that can help stop pain at the originating point, which is usually along the lower spine rather than in the buttocks, hips, or legs, where cramping is occurring. Using your fingertips, apply 3 or 4 drops of bergamot essential oil directly to the lower spine, following it with a few drops of carrier oil to prevent irritation at the site. Repeat this treatment once a day as needed, following a good stretch and a hot bath.

ROSEMARY-PEPPERMINT MASSAGE OIL

MAKES 1 TREATMENT

Rosemary, peppermint, and eucalyptus essential oils penetrate deep into tissue to relax muscles and ease pain. Stretch before applying this massage oil, and make it even more effective by taking a hot bath prior to application.

1 tablespoon carrier oil
4 drops rosemary essential oil
3 drops peppermint essential oil
2 drops eucalyptus essential oil

1. In a small glass bowl, add the carrier oil along with the rosemary, peppermint, and eucalyptus essential oils, and stir to combine.
2. Using your fingertips, apply the blend to the lower back, buttocks, and hips, and massage it into the skin, taking care to avoid the anus, as these essential oils can cause stinging. Rub with moderate pressure, using long, firm strokes.
3. Repeat this treatment up to 2 times a day until symptoms subside.

Seasonal Affective Disorder (SAD)

Seasonal affective disorder (SAD) usually begins as days shorten in fall or winter, and ends as days grow longer during spring and summer. The feelings of sadness, tiredness, and depression that often accompany SAD are caused by reduced serotonin production. Essential oils and light therapy can turn SAD around in most cases. If these treatments do not work, seek medical intervention.

MELISSA-ORANGE SMELLING SALTS

MAKES 1 TREATMENT

Melissa, orange, and peppermint essential oils uplift the spirits and help restore balance on dark, gloomy winter days.

1 tablespoon sea salt
6 drops melissa essential oil
6 drops orange essential oil
6 drops peppermint essential oil

1. In a dark-colored glass bottle, add the sea salt along with the melissa, orange, and peppermint essential oils, and shake well to blend.
2. Inhale the blend when feeling low, or leave it uncapped next to you.
3. Repeat this treatment as needed. Refresh the blend periodically by adding more melissa, orange, and peppermint essential oil.

YLANG-YLANG BATH OIL

MAKES 1 TREATMENT

Ylang-ylang essential oil is among the best natural antidepressants available, easing worry and anxiety while leaving a peaceful, euphoric feeling behind. Use ylang-ylang as much as you like, and try different therapies that incorporate the essential oil. It is wonderful for diffusing in your home or carrying with you in an aromatherapy pendant.

1 tablespoon carrier oil
6 drops ylang-ylang essential oil

1. In a small glass bowl, add the carrier oil and ylang-ylang essential oil, and stir to combine.
2. Draw a warm bath and add the entire treatment to the running water.
3. Soak for at least 15 minutes. Use caution when getting out of the bathtub, as it may be slippery.
4. Repeat this treatment once a day as needed.

Shingles

Shingles happen when the chicken pox virus reactivates. Symptoms include sensitivity to light, headache, and flu-like symptoms without fever. Itching, pain, and tingling also occur, along with a small, painful rash that forms blisters before scabbing over. While essential oils often bring comfort in mild cases of shingles, medical treatment is required in severe cases.

NEAT CLOVE TREATMENT

Clove essential oil helps stop the virus that causes shingles while numbing the itching and pain experienced during an outbreak. Using a cotton swab or a spray bottle, apply a small amount of clove essential oil to each affected area. Repeat this treatment as needed until the shingles outbreak subsides.

ROSE GERANIUM SALVE

MAKES 1 TREATMENT

Rose geranium soothes itching and burning while helping skin recover from trauma. Use geranium essential oil if you do not have rose geranium essential oil.

1 teaspoon carrier oil
8 drops rose geranium essential oil

1. In a small glass bowl, add the carrier oil and rose geranium essential oil, and stir to combine.
2. Using your fingertips, apply the blend to affected area.
3. Repeat this treatment up to 3 times a day until the shingles outbreak subsides.

Shin Splints

Shin splints are characterized by sore, throbbing shins. Caused by overuse, swollen or irritated muscles, and even tiny stress fractures in the lower leg bones, shin splints often heal on their own. Rest, elevation, ice, and essential oils can help. If symptoms do not start to subside within three days, contact your doctor. You may have serious stress fractures that require surgery.

HELICHRYSUM-LEMONGRASS MASSAGE

MAKES 1 TREATMENT

Helichrysum, lemongrass, and myrrh essential oils penetrate to help injured tissue heal faster than when left untreated. They also ease the pain somewhat. Use a hot compress to cover your shins after this treatment for even more relief.

1 tablespoon carrier oil
10 drops helichrysum essential oil
10 drops lemongrass essential oil
10 drops myrrh essential oil

1. In a small glass bowl, add the carrier oil along with the helichrysum, lemongrass, and myrrh essential oils, and stir to combine.
2. Using your fingertips, apply the blend to the shins, and massage it into the skin using medium pressure and long, even strokes.
3. Repeat this treatment up to 6 times a day until symptoms subside.

PEPPERMINT ICE

MAKES 1 TREATMENT

Peppermint essential oil penetrates tissue, helping temporarily stop pain. Placing an ice pack on top intensifies the feeling of relief while alleviating inflammation.

10 drops peppermint essential oil
1 ice pack

1. Using your fingertips, apply the peppermint essential oil directly to the shin, then top it with a towel.
2. Place the ice pack on top of the towel and leave in place for at least 10 minutes but no more than 20 minutes.
3. Repeat this treatment once an hour until the pain subsides. If both legs are affected, alternate the treatment on each leg.

Sinusitis

Sinusitis is inflammation or an infection of the mucus membranes lining the sinuses and inner nasal passages. Caused by bacteria, fungi, or viruses, sinusitis is characterized by symptoms that include blocked nasal passages, a headache, fever, dental pain, reduced sense of smell or taste, bad breath, and a cough that produces mucus. Essential oils can help ease symptoms, which should go away within 10 to 14 days. See your doctor if your condition becomes worse instead of improving.

CAJEPUT BATH

MAKES 1 TREATMENT

Cajeput essential oil is a strong antiseptic that helps combat sinusitis, particularly when steam vapor is inhaled.

1 tablespoon carrier oil
6 drops cajeput essential oil

1. In a small glass bowl, add the carrier oil and cajeput essential oil, and stir to combine.
2. Draw a warm bath and add the entire treatment to the running water.
3. Soak for at least 15 minutes. Use caution when getting out of the bathtub, as it may be slippery.
4. Repeat this treatment once a day until symptoms subside.

FOUR-OIL BLEND SINUS RELIEF

MAKES 1 TREATMENT

Peppermint, rosemary, eucalyptus, and thyme essential oils alleviate sinus pressure and inflammation while opening the airway.

3 cups hot water
2 drops peppermint essential oil
2 drops rosemary essential oil
1 drop eucalyptus essential oil
1 drop thyme essential oil

1. In a medium glass bowl, add the hot water along with the peppermint, rosemary, eucalyptus, and thyme essential oils, and stir to combine.
2. Sit comfortably, tenting your head with a towel over the bowl, and breathe deeply for 5 minutes, emerging for fresh air as needed.
3. Repeat this treatment as needed until symptoms subside.

Skin Tags

Skin tags are a primarily cosmetic concern. These small flaps hang from the skin via a slender connecting stalk; they are skin-colored and are normally painless, although they can become irritated if they rub against clothing or jewelry. If essential oils do not help, you can have your doctor remove your skin tag for you by freezing it with liquid nitrogen, burning it off, or removing it with a scalpel.

ELIMINATE WITH FRANKINCENSE

Frankincense essential oil can be applied directly to skin tags, particularly if they are sore and inflamed. Apply 1 drop of essential oil to each skin tag. Repeat this treatment 2 times a day until the skin tags are gone. This treatment works best on smaller skin tags; larger ones respond better to treatment with tea tree essential oil.

BANISH WITH TEA TREE

Tea tree essential oil has a strong drying effect that skin tags normally can't resist. Apply 1 drop of tea tree essential oil to each skin tag. Repeat this treatment 2 times a day until the skin tags are gone.

Slow Metabolism

Lose excess weight and increase your energy level by boosting your metabolism naturally. These remedies work best when paired with a sensible diet and increased physical activity. In some cases, poor metabolism can be indicative of an underlying medical problem. If a healthy diet, regular exercise, and treatment with natural remedies fail to make a noticeable difference within a few months, consult your doctor.

FRUITY HERBAL BATH

MAKES 7 TREATMENTS

You can reap the metabolic rewards grapefruit essential oil has to offer in a relaxing bath, while reflecting on more ways you can be good to yourself.

16 drops grapefruit essential oil
9 drops basil essential oil
9 drops cypress essential oil
9 drops lavender essential oil
6 drops juniper essential oil

1. In a dark-colored glass bottle, add the grapefruit, basil, cypress, lavender, and juniper essential oils, and shake well to blend.
2. Draw a warm bath and add 7 drops of the essential oil blend to the running water.
3. Soak for at least 15 minutes. Use caution when getting out of the bathtub, as it may be slippery.
4. Repeat this treatment once a day.

Smoking Cessation

Quitting tobacco is among the best things you can do for your overall health. Stress can often feel overwhelming during this time, and using essential oils to keep it under control can help eliminate the temptation to resume your habit.

STOP CRAVINGS WITH BLACK PEPPER

Black pepper essential oil helps increase energy and dispel stress while helping eliminate tobacco cravings. Diffuse black pepper essential oil in the area where you spend the most time, add it to an aromatherapy pendant, or simply place 2 or 3 drops on a cotton ball near you. Repeat this treatment each time you feel the urge to use tobacco.

Sore Throat

A sore throat often begins with a feeling of itchiness just behind the roof of the mouth; redness, irritation, and pain often follow. Additional symptoms include difficulty swallowing and speaking. Sore throats normally accompany other illnesses; they are not typically cause for concern unless other symptoms are severe or debilitating.

CAJEPUT CHEST MASSAGE

MAKES 1 TREATMENT

Cajeput essential oil is a strong antiseptic with the ability to help alleviate a sore throat, particularly when inhaled or used topically. By using a chest massage, you benefit both ways.

1 teaspoon carrier oil
4 drops cajeput essential oil

1. Using your fingertips, apply the carrier oil to the chest, followed by the cajeput essential oil.
2. Cover the chest with a T-shirt or cloth, relax, and breathe deeply.
3. Repeat this treatment as needed until symptoms subside.

GERANIUM-HYSSOP GARGLE

MAKES 1 TREATMENT

Geranium and hyssop essential oils ease pain and inflammation while promoting recovery and helping stop bacteria from growing out of control.

1 ounce purified water
3 drops geranium essential oil
3 drops hyssop essential oil

1. In a small drinking glass, add the water along with the geranium and hyssop essential oils, and stir to combine.
2. Gargle with the solution for as long as you can.
3. Repeat this treatment as needed until symptoms subside.

Spider Bites

Spider bites are often itchy, swollen, and slightly painful. Refrain from scratching during treatment, as this can cause the venom to spread and increase your discomfort. Seek emergency treatment if you have been bitten by a poisonous spider such as a brown recluse or black widow.

NEAT LAVENDER TREATMENT

Lavender essential oil aids in detoxification while helping stop the pain and itching associated with spider bites. Using your fingertips, apply 1 drop of lavender essential oil to the bite as soon after it occurs as possible. Repeat this treatment every 1 to 2 hours until the pain and itching subside.

NEAT BASIL TREATMENT

Basil essential oil has a numbing effect that stops pain and itching; it also helps soothe inflammation. Using your fingertips, apply 1 drop of basil essential oil to the bite as soon after it occurs as possible. Repeat this treatment every 1 to 2 hours until the pain and itching subside.

Sprain

Sprains are stretched or torn ligaments that normally occur when a joint is twisted or hit in a way that forces it out of its normal position. Minor sprains respond very well to treatment at home; essential oils, ice, rest, elevation, and compression help ease the pain. If you heard a cracking noise at the time of injury or if swelling, pain, or discoloration is severe, see your doctor for an X-ray. You should also see your doctor even if an affected limb is not a weight-bearing limb.

PEPPERMINT COMPRESS

MAKES 1 TREATMENT

Peppermint essential oil penetrates deep into tissue to temporarily stop pain. Using it in concert with a cold compress can help alleviate pain while keeping swelling to a minimum.

Peppermint essential oil
1 pint cold water

1. Using your fingertips, apply peppermint essential oil to the sprained area, using as much as is required to thinly coat the sprain.
2. In a medium glass bowl, add the cold water.
3. Submerge a towel in the water, wring it out, apply the compress to the affected area, and elevate the sprained limb. Leave the compress in place until it warms to body temperature.
4. Repeat this treatment every 1 to 2 hours during the first day of the injury, and repeat this treatment as needed thereafter.

THYME SALVE

MAKES 1 TREATMENT

Thyme essential oil is both an analgesic and an anti-inflammatory, making it the ideal remedy for soothing sprains.

1 teaspoon carrier oil
8 drops thyme essential oil

1. Using your fingertips, apply the carrier oil to the affected area, followed by the thyme essential oil.
2. Elevate the sprained limb and rest for at least 15 minutes.
3. Repeat this treatment up to 3 times a day until the pain and inflammation subside.

Stiff Neck

Neck stiffness might happen during a long drive or after an extended work session spent sitting at your desk, staring at your computer. Essential oils often bring prompt relief and promote relaxation. If the cause of your neck stiffness is not apparent and it continues or worsens, or is accompanied by a fever or nausea, contact your doctor, as there may be a serious underlying illness present.

CLARY SAGE-LAVANDIN SALVE

MAKES 1 TREATMENT

Clary sage and lavandin essential oils relax the mind and soothe tired, sore muscles while helping alleviate stress and put you in a positive frame of mind.

1/2 teaspoon carrier oil
4 drops clary sage essential oil
3 drops lavandin essential oil

1. In a small glass bowl, add the carrier oil along with the clary sage and lavandin essential oils, and stir to combine.
2. Using your fingertips, apply the blend to the neck and shoulder area, and massage it into the skin. Stretch your neck from side to side, then relax.
3. Repeat this treatment up to 4 times a day as needed.

ROSEMARY SALVE

MAKES 1 TREATMENT

Rosemary essential oil penetrates deep into sore muscles, helping alleviate stiffness. It also invigorates and refreshes the mind while helping you relax.

½ teaspoon carrier oil
4 drops rosemary essential oil

1. In a small glass bowl, add the carrier oil and rosemary essential oil, and stir to combine.
2. Using your fingertips, apply the blend to the neck and shoulders, and massage it into the skin. Stretch your neck from side to side and relax.
3. Repeat this treatment up to 6 times a day as needed.

Stomach Flu

With nausea, vomiting, diarrhea, and the inability to hold down food, stomach flu is a miserable illness. Also known as gastroenteritis and not associated with the flu virus, the stomach flu usually lasts from 24 to 48 hours, although you may not feel like yourself again for up to a week. Call your doctor if you have severe diarrhea that lasts for two days or longer, if vomiting lasts for more than one day, if you are pregnant, or if your stools have a black, tarry appearance or are streaked with blood.

HYSSOP BATH

MAKES 1 TREATMENT

Hyssop essential oil helps stop nausea and vomiting, and it relaxes and soothes the mind so you can rest. This bath allows you to benefit from vapors as well as absorption.

1 tablespoon carrier oil
6 drops hyssop essential oil

1. In a small glass bowl, add the carrier oil and hyssop essential oil, and stir to combine.
2. Draw a warm bath and add the entire treatment to the running water.
3. Soak for at least 15 minutes. Use caution when getting out of the bathtub, as it may be slippery.

Strep Throat

Strep throat is a painful bacterial infection of the throat and tonsils that is highly contagious. The most common symptoms of strep throat are swollen tonsils and lymph nodes, a fever over 101 degrees Fahrenheit, and yellow or white spots in the back of the throat. Cold symptoms like coughing, a runny nose, and sneezing do not normally accompany strep throat. While essential oils can ease your symptoms, antibiotics are normally recommended. Without a prescription, you may remain contagious for as long as three weeks, even if your symptoms have disappeared completely.

RELAXING LEMON-ROSEWOOD BATH

MAKES 1 TREATMENT

Lemon and rosewood essential oils help stop infection while addressing uncomfortable strep throat symptoms. You can diffuse a blend of equal amounts of the two essential oils in the room you're occupying while sick, in addition to enjoying this bath.

1 tablespoon carrier oil
5 drops rosewood essential oil
2 drops lemon essential oil

1. In a small glass bowl, add the carrier oil along with the rosewood and lemon essential oils, and stir to combine.
2. Draw a warm bath and add the entire treatment to the running water.
3. Soak for at least 15 minutes. Use caution when getting out of the bathtub, as it may be slippery.
4. Repeat this treatment 4 times a day as needed.

SANDALWOOD GARGLE

MAKES 1 TREATMENT

Sandalwood essential oil helps stop infection while soothing pain. You can also benefit by using it in the bathtub or shower. If you do not have sandalwood essential oil, make this gargle with tea tree essential oil instead.

1 ounce water
4 drops sandalwood essential oil

1. In a drinking glass, add the water and sandalwood essential oil, and stir to combine.
2. Gargle for at least 15 seconds.
3. Repeat this treatment as needed until symptoms subside.

Stress Management

Stress can lead to or complicate other health disorders, so keeping the stressors of daily life from becoming overwhelming should be among your chief concerns. Essential oils help mitigate stress, as do exercise, rest, and a healthy, natural diet.

DIFFUSE ALLSPICE

Allspice essential oil, also know as pimento essential oil, is exceptional for alleviating stress and warding off feelings of overwhelmed inadequacy. Diffuse allspice essential oil in the area where you spend the most time, or carry it with you in an aromatherapy pendant. A few drops can be added to your bath or to a washcloth placed on the floor of your shower, too.

CLARY SAGE-TANGERINE SMELLING SALTS

MAKES 1 TREATMENT

Both clary sage and tangerine essential oils have the ability to help you stay alert and focused so you can accomplish the things you need to get done. Use these smelling salts anytime you feel overwhelmed.

1 tablespoon sea salt
6 drops clary sage essential oil
2 drops tangerine essential oil

1. In a dark-colored glass bottle, add the sea salt along with the clary sage and tangerine essential oils, and shake well to blend.
2. Inhale the blend.
3. Repeat this treatment as needed. Refresh the salts periodically by adding more clary sage and tangerine essential oils.

Stretch Marks

Stretch marks are usually associated with pregnancy, but they can also occur with sudden weight gain, rapid increases in muscle mass, and Cushing's disease. Stretch marks are scars that begin as reddish to purplish lines before eventually losing their color. Stretch marks are primarily of cosmetic concern; if essential oils don't work, a dermatologist may be able to remove them via surgical methods.

NEAT HELICHRYSUM TREATMENT

Helichrysum essential oil improves skin's elasticity while rapidly healing damaged tissue. This remedy is most effective on new stretch marks, and if treated early on, you may be able to eliminate them completely. Using this essential oil may fade older stretch marks if they are not serious; however, do not be surprised if only a small change occurs. Using your fingertips, apply the helichrysum essential oil liberally to new stretch marks once a day until satisfied.

JASMINE-MANDARIN MASSAGE

MAKES 1 TREATMENT

Jasmine and mandarin essential oils help damaged tissue heal while softening and smoothing surrounding tissue.

1 tablespoon carrier oil
6 drops jasmine essential oil
2 drops mandarin essential oil

1. In a small glass bowl, add the carrier oil along with the jasmine and mandarin essential oils, and stir to combine.
2. Using your fingertips, apply the blend liberally to new stretch marks.
3. Repeat this treatment once a day until you are satisfied with the results.

Sunburn

A sunburn occurs when the sun's ultraviolet rays penetrate the skin, causing pain and redness. While it is best to prevent sunburns by limiting exposure to the sun, it is a common problem that can be difficult to avoid. Seek medical treatment if swelling and severe pain occur or if a fever is present. In some cases, skin infections occur following severe sunburns, necessitating medical intervention.

COOLING PEPPERMINT SPRAY

MAKES 24 TREATMENTS

Peppermint essential oil helps cool sunburns while acting as a mild analgesic. This spray should not be used on blistered skin.

4 ounces water
10 drops peppermint essential oil

1. In a dark-colored glass bottle fitted with a spray top, add the water and peppermint essential oil, and shake well to blend.
2. Spray the blend on the affected area and allow it to air-dry before putting on clothes.
3. Repeat this treatment as needed until the sunburn fades. Shake the bottle before each use.

SOOTHING LAVENDER-TEA TREE SPRITZ

MAKES 24 TREATMENTS

Lavender and tea tree essential oils help stop sunburn pain while treating compromised skin. Use this treatment as soon as possible following a sunburn for best results.

4 ounces water
30 drops lavender essential oil
20 drops tea tree essential oil

1. In a dark-colored glass bottle fitted with a spray top, add the water along with the lavender and tea tree essential oils, and shake well to blend.
2. Spray the blend on the affected area and allow it to air-dry before putting on clothes.
3. Repeat this treatment as needed until the sunburn fades. Shake the bottle before each use.

Swelling

Swelling is characterized by an increase in the size of a body part; in some cases, the shape of the body part may change dramatically, as well. Swelling usually accompanies other illnesses; even so, essential oils may help stop the discomfort. Seek medical attention if you're not sure what caused the swelling, or if the swelling is accompanied by extreme pain. In addition, you should seek emergency treatment if severe swelling is present after an injury of any kind, as an underlying fracture could be present.

FENNEL-CYPRESS MASSAGE

MAKES 1 TREATMENT

Fennel and cypress help soothe inflammation while acting as a diuretic to draw excess fluid away from swollen tissue.

1 tablespoon carrier oil
15 drops fennel essential oil
10 drops cypress essential oil

1. In a small glass bowl, add the carrier oil along with the fennel and cypress essential oils, and stir to combine.
2. Using your fingertips, apply the blend to the affected area, and massage it into the skin, working your way toward your heart.
3. Repeat this treatment every 2 to 3 hours as needed.

GRAPEFRUIT-LEMONGRASS SALVE

MAKES 1 TREATMENT

Grapefruit and lemongrass essential oils act as diuretics to help alleviate swelling, and grape seed oil helps strengthen tissue to prevent damage.

1 tablespoon grape seed carrier oil
6 drops grapefruit essential oil
4 drops lemongrass essential oil

1. In a small glass bowl, add the grape seed carrier oil along with the grapefruit and lemongrass essential oils, and stir to combine.
2. Using your fingertips, apply the blend to the affected area, and massage it into the skin, working your way toward your heart.
3. Repeat this treatment every 2 to 3 hours as needed.

Swimmer's Ear

Swimmer's ear is an infection or inflammation of the ear canal, which is the passage leading from the outer portion of the ear to the eardrum. Caused by fungal or bacterial growth in the ear canal, swimmer's ear brings itching, pain, and redness with it. See your doctor if brown or yellow discharge is emerging from the ear or if extreme pain and swelling are present. If you take medication that suppresses your immune system or if you are diabetic, see your doctor immediately, since swimmer's ear can cause severe complications.

NEAT TEA TREE TREATMENT

Tea tree essential oil helps dry swimmer's ear while killing bacteria. Place a cotton ball that has been treated with 4 or 5 drops of tea tree essential oil into the ear and leave it in place overnight. Apply this treatment at the first sign of irritation for fast relief. Repeat this treatment as needed until the irritation is gone.

NEAT BASIL TREATMENT

Basil essential oil stops bacteria while helping ease discomfort. Place a cotton ball that has been treated with 4 or 5 drops of basil essential oil into the ear and leave it in place overnight. Apply this treatment at the first sign of irritation for fast relief. Repeat this treatment as needed until the irritation is gone.

Teething

As a baby's primary teeth erupt, swelling, redness, itching, and pain are often present. Babies who are teething often cry, sometimes inconsolably. Essential oils can soothe the pain and ease the stress that comes with teething.

CLOVE TEETHING SALVE

MAKES 24 TREATMENTS

Clove essential oil is a strong analgesic that helps stop the pain of teething. It must be heavily diluted for use in babies.

2 tablespoons olive carrier oil
2 drops clove essential oil

1. In a small glass bowl, add the olive carrier oil and clove essential oil, and stir to combine.
2. Test a dot of the blend on your own gums to be sure you can feel the clove but that the mixture is not too spicy; adjust with more clove essential oil or additional olive carrier oil if needed.
3. Using your fingertips, apply the blend sparingly to the child's gums.
4. Repeat this treatment every 1 to 2 hours as needed.

GRAPEFRUIT TEETHING SALVE

MAKES 1 TREATMENT

Grapefruit essential oil is an effective analgesic that's milder than clove essential oil. Diffuse some lavender essential oil in your home to promote calm and supplement teething remedies.

3 drops olive carrier oil
1 drop grapefruit essential oil

1. In a small glass bowl, add the carrier oil and grapefruit essential oil, and stir to combine.
2. Using your fingertips, apply the blend sparingly to the child's gums.
3. Repeat this treatment every 1 to 2 hours as needed.

Temper Tantrums

Temper tantrums aren't bad behavior on your child's part. Instead, these outbursts are unplanned, unintentional displays of frustration and anger that happen, usually when a child is overtired. While preventing or eliminating triggers can go a long way, essential oils can help calm a stressed child. If your child bites, hits, or kicks you or others during temper tantrums, an underlying psychological problem could be to blame. Seek professional help if your child frequently expresses uncontrollable rage.

DIFFUSE YLANG-YLANG

Ylang-ylang essential oil helps the mind deal with disruptive emotions, replacing feelings of stress, frustration, and anger with relaxed calm. Diffuse ylang-ylang essential oil in the room where the child is having the tantrum. If you don't have a diffuser, make a simple room spray by combining 4 ounces of water with 24 drops of ylang-ylang essential oil. Use it as needed at home, in the car, and wherever you and your little one spend time.

ROSE TEDDY BEAR

MAKES 1 TREATMENT

Rose essential oil soothes fear, eases nervous tension, alleviates stress, and helps the mind cope with unruly emotions.

1 favorite stuffed animal
2 drops rose essential oil

1. Dab the essential oil onto the stuffed animal and give it to the child.
2. Repeat this treatment as needed to promote a calm, harmonious home.

Tendinitis

Tendons are thick, strong tissues that connect muscles with bones. When they become inflamed, the result is tendinitis—a painful or tender condition that is often accompanied by stiffness and mild swelling. Rest, hot and cold therapy, and essential oils are usually enough to ease the pain. Call your doctor if there is no improvement within 10 days. In addition, seek emergency treatment if severe pain with swelling and reduced range of motion is present; you may have a ruptured tendon, in which case surgical intervention may be necessary.

MARJORAM COMPRESS

Marjoram essential oil penetrates deep into sore, inflamed tissue, stopping pain and promoting relaxation. Using a warm compress atop the essential oil helps drive it deeper into tissue.

1 teaspoon carrier oil
6 drops marjoram essential oil
1 pint hot water

1. Using your fingertips, apply the carrier oil to the affected area, followed by the marjoram essential oil.
2. In a medium glass bowl, add the hot water.
3. Submerge a towel in the water, wring it out, and apply the compress to the affected area. Layer plastic wrap on top of the compress to keep the essential oil vapors from evaporating. Leave the compress in place until it cools to body temperature.
4. Repeat this treatment as needed.

COOLING EUCALYPTUS-PEPPERMINT RUB

MAKES 1 TREATMENT

Eucalyptus and peppermint essential oils stop pain while promoting relaxation. The cooling sensation this remedy provides is pleasant, and its aroma is uplifting.

1 teaspoon carrier oil
4 drops eucalyptus essential oil
4 drops peppermint essential oil

1. In a small glass bowl, add the carrier oil along with the eucalyptus and peppermint essential oils, and stir to combine.
2. Using your fingertips, apply the blend to the affected area, and massage it into the skin.
3. Repeat this treatment every 2 to 3 hours as needed, adding carrier oil between treatments to prevent the skin from drying.

Tennis Elbow

Tennis elbow is so named because it's common among tennis players, but any overuse of the hand, arm, and forearm muscles can contribute to the problem. Characterized by pain and stiffness at the point where the forearm's muscles connect to the bony portion of the outer elbow, this injury usually calls for medical intervention. Use essential oils to help keep discomfort to a minimum while recovering.

MARJORAM RUBDOWN

Marjoram essential oil penetrates deep into tissue, stopping pain and promoting relaxation. Using your fingertips, apply 2 or 3 drops of marjoram essential oil to the affected area, and massage it into the skin. Add a bit more essential oil if additional relief from pain is still needed. Repeat this treatment every 2 to 3 hours as needed, adding carrier oil between treatments to prevent the skin from drying.

NUTMEG SALVE

MAKES 1 TREATMENT

Nutmeg essential oil penetrates deep into tissue, stopping pain and aiding in relaxation while improving circulation. Its fragrance helps lift the spirits; most people find it quite pleasant.

½ teaspoon carrier oil
2 drops nutmeg essential oil

1. In a small glass bowl, add the carrier oil and nutmeg essential oils, and stir to combine.
2. Using your fingertips, apply the blend to the affected area, and massage it into the skin.
3. Repeat this treatment every 2 to 3 hours as needed.

Tension Headache

Usually brought on by stress, tension headaches can also be triggered by depression, muscle strain, or hunger. Most last for only a short time, but some last for as long as seven days. Essential oils can help soothe the pain and stress associated with tension headaches; you may discover that they work just as well as or better than OTC pain remedies. Consult your doctor if you suffer from chronic headaches, as they can be symptomatic of an underlying illness.

PEPPERMINT TEMPLE RUB

Peppermint essential oil stops pain and soothes tension. For mild headaches, rubbing the temples with 1 drop of peppermint essential oil per side is often enough to have an almost immediate effect. For stronger headaches, apply the essential oil to the temples, and use 3 to 5 drops on the back of the neck, as well.

THREE-OIL RELAXATION COMPRESS

MAKES 1 TREATMENT

Frankincense, lavender, and peppermint essential oils soothe headaches by promoting relaxation and interfering with the body's pain signals. Applying a cool compress helps speed relief.

3 drops frankincense essential oil
3 drops lavender essential oil
3 drops peppermint essential oil
1 pint cold water

1. In the palm of your hand, add the frankincense, lavender, and peppermint essential oils.
2. Rub your hands together, then cup them over your mouth and inhale 3 to 5 times.
3. Rub the essential oils onto your forehead.
4. In a medium glass bowl, add the cold water.
5. Submerge a towel in the water, wring it out, and apply the compress to the forehead, taking care to prevent water and essential oils from dripping into your eyes. Leave the compress in place until it warms to body temperature.
6. Repeat this treatment every 2 to 3 hours as needed.

Thrush

Thrush can affect anyone, but it is most common in babies and elderly people. It is caused when a type of yeast called candida grows out of control and is exacerbated by a weak immune system. Thrush brings itching, pain, and white patches that look a bit like cottage cheese. Give essential oils 2 to 3 days to work; if thrush does not improve or gets worse, contact your doctor.

TEA TREE SPRAY

MAKES 24 TREATMENTS

Tea tree essential oil stops discomfort while eliminating the fungus that causes thrush.

4 ounces water
6 drops tea tree essential oil

1. In a dark-colored glass bottle fitted with a spray top, add the water and tea tree essential oil, and shake well to blend.
2. Spray the inside of the mouth. For young babies, you may need to apply the spray to a cloth and gently wipe the inside of the mouth.
3. Repeat this treatment 2 to 4 times a day until symptoms subside.

Tick Bites

Unlike other insects, ticks fasten themselves to the skin, where they feed on blood for an extended period of time. Most ticks do not carry disease, and at most, you will probably experience redness and irritation after a bite. Monitor your health following a tick bite, as tick-borne illnesses can take several weeks to manifest. If you believe you have contracted a tick-borne illness, contact your doctor immediately, as life-threatening complications can develop.

NEAT NIAOULI TREATMENT

Niaouli essential oil stops the stinging and itching that can accompany a tick bite while helping prevent infection and inflammation. Using your fingertips, apply 1 drop of niaouli essential oil to the affected area after the tick has been removed. Repeat this treatment as needed until the irritation subsides.

NEAT TEA TREE TREATMENT

Tea tree essential oil stops the itching and swelling that can accompany a tick bite while helping prevent infection and inflammation. Using your fingertips, apply 1 drop of tea tree essential oil to the affected area after the tick has been removed. Repeat this treatment as needed until irritation subsides.

Tinnitus

Tinnitus, or ringing in the ears, can be a symptom of an underlying illness, or it may be caused by something as simple as built-up earwax. Often, tinnitus goes away by itself within a few days. If your symptoms last for more than two weeks, or if you have a fever or ear drainage, see your doctor. You should also seek treatment if tinnitus happens right after a head injury occurs.

NEAT HELICHRYSUM TREATMENT

Helichrysum essential oil stops inflammation and may help ease tinnitus symptoms. Apply 1 drop of helichrysum essential oil on each of 2 cotton balls. Place 1 cotton ball in each ear and leave them in place for up to 2 hours. Repeat this treatment as needed.

BASIL-FRANKINCENSE SALVE

MAKES 1 TREATMENT

Basil and frankincense essential oils penetrate the ears and help stop discomfort associated with tinnitus. Their fragrances help ease anxiety and stress, which may in turn help speed relief.

2 drops basil essential oil
2 drops frankincense essential oil

1. In the palm of your hand, add the basil and frankincense essential oils.
2. Using your fingertips, apply the blend to the backs of your ears and to the portion of your jaw line directly beneath the ears.
3. Repeat this treatment every 2 to 3 hours until the ringing subsides.

Toothache

Toothaches happen for a number of reasons, including trauma, infection, and inflammation. Pain may be dull and throbbing, or sharp and unbearable. Sensitivity to heat and cold as well as pain when chewing are common, and swollen or bleeding gums around the tooth may also occur. Call your doctor or dentist if remedies do not relieve the pain within 24 hours or if a tooth has been broken or knocked out. If you have dental pain that is radiating to your jawbone, seek treatment right away, as a serious infection could be present.

NEAT CLOVE TREATMENT

Clove essential oil numbs even sharp tooth pain and can serve as a suitable first-aid measure until your dental appointment in the event you have a serious problem. Using your fingertips, apply 1 drop of clove essential oil to the affected tooth and surrounding tissue, breathing through your mouth for 1 to 2 minutes to allow it to penetrate. Repeat this treatment every 2 to 3 hours as needed.

CHEEK MASSAGE

MAKES 1 TREATMENT

German chamomile, clove, and lemon essential oils come together to bring pain relief and reduce inflammation when a toothache causes facial pain.

1 teaspoon carrier oil
3 drops German chamomile essential oil
2 drops clove essential oil
2 drops lemon essential oil

1. In a small glass bowl, add the carrier oil along with the German chamomile, clove, and lemon essential oils, and stir to combine.
2. Using your fingertips, apply the blend to the cheek and jaw area, and massage it gently into the affected area.
3. Repeat this treatment every 2 to 3 hours as needed.

Urinary Tract Infection

The need to urinate urgently and frequently, pain or irritation when urinating, and cloudy or smelly urine are among the symptoms of a urinary tract infection. It's vital to address this condition immediately if you hope to treat it with essential oils. If the pain worsens or if a fever develops, contact your doctor. In addition, you should call your doctor if you are pregnant, over 65, or have diabetes, a weak immune system, or kidney problems.

BERGAMOT MASSAGE

MAKES 1 TREATMENT

Bergamot essential oil has strong antibiotic and antiseptic properties. It is easily absorbed into the body via massage. Use a warm compress after the massage for extra relief.

1 tablespoon carrier oil
6 drops bergamot essential oil

1. In a small glass bowl, add the carrier oil and bergamot essential oil, and stir to combine.
2. Using your fingertips, apply the blend to the lower abdomen area, and massage it into the skin.
3. Repeat this treatment 2 to 4 times a day for 4 days. However, if symptoms worsen after 1 day, stop this treatment and see a doctor.

CEDARWOOD COMPRESS

MAKES 1 TREATMENT

Cedarwood essential oil is a strong antiseptic that sometimes helps stop urinary tract infections. It is not safe for ingestion and should be kept away from mucus membranes.

6 drops cedarwood essential oil
1 teaspoon carrier oil
1 pint hot water

1. Using your fingertips, apply the cedarwood essential oil to your lower abdomen, followed by the carrier oil.
2. In a medium bowl, add the hot water.
3. Submerge a towel in the water, wring it out, and apply the compress to the affected area. Leave the compress in place until it cools to body temperature.
4. Repeat this treatment as needed.

Varicose Veins

Varicose veins and spider veins can be seen through the skin, usually as blue to purple blood vessels that appear to be swollen. Aching, tiredness, throbbing, and tingling are common symptoms; wearing support hose, elevating the legs, and treating with essential oils can provide relief, as can lifestyle changes. While these treatments are not likely to make varicose veins disappear, they ease symptoms. Medical intervention is not normally necessary, although there are effective treatments for removing varicose veins altogether.

CYPRESS-LAVENDER RUB

MAKES 1 TREATMENT

Cypress and lavender essential oils combine to alleviate the inflammation and pain that accompany varicose veins.

1 tablespoon carrier oil
4 drops cypress essential oil
4 drops lavender essential oil

1. In a small glass bowl, add the carrier oil along with the cypress and lavender essential oils, and stir to combine.
2. Using your fingertips, apply the blend to the affected areas, and massage it into the skin, working toward the heart.
3. Repeat the treatment up to 4 times a day as needed.

GERANIUM-CYPRESS MASSAGE

MAKES 1 TREATMENT

Geranium and cypress essential oils combine to ease discomfort and inflammation associated with varicose veins while promoting healthy circulation. Remember to elevate your legs frequently to help prevent swelling. This blend is fantastic in baths, as well.

1 tablespoon carrier oil
8 drops geranium essential oil
3 drops cypress essential oil

1. In a small glass bowl, add the carrier oil along with the geranium and cypress essential oils, and stir to combine.
2. Using your fingertips, apply the blend to the affected areas, and massage it into the skin, working toward the heart.
3. Repeat the treatment up to 4 times a day as needed.

Warts

Warts are bumpy, rough, or hardened areas of skin that grow faster than the surrounding skin. Most warts are harmless; however, the virus that causes them is highly contagious. Contact your doctor if you have genital warts, or if you are not certain that a skin growth is a wart, or if symptoms of infection such as pain, pus, redness, fever, or swelling are present.

REMOVE WITH TEA TREE

Tea tree essential oil is one of the most effective natural wart removal remedies available. Using your fingertips, apply 1 drop of tea tree essential oil to the surface of the wart and let it dry. Repeat this treatment up to 3 times a day until the wart fades.

CYPRESS-LAVENDER-LEMON WART REMOVER

MAKES 24 TREATMENTS

Cypress, lavender, and lemon essential oils help dry out warts and stop the virus that causes them. This blend is intended for people over 12 years old. Dilute the blend in equal amounts with a carrier oil for younger children.

8 drops cypress essential oil
8 drops lavender essential oil
8 drops lemon essential oil

1. In a dark-colored glass bottle, add the cypress, lavender, and lemon essential oils, and shake well to blend.
2. Using your fingertips, apply 1 drop of the blend to the wart.
3. Repeat this treatment 2 times a day until the wart fades.

Wasp Stings

Essential oils are a great natural way to treat wasp stings or prevent them from happening by repelling wasps. With essential oils, you can avoid the commercial wasp repellents that are laden with toxic chemicals that can harm you, your children, your pets, and the environment.

WASP REPELLENT

MAKES 24 TREATMENTS

Wasps often seem to arrive just as you're sitting down to a picnic. Thyme essential oil emits vapors that drive them away.

4 ounces water
24 drops thyme essential oil

1. In a dark-colored glass bottle fitted with a spray top, add the water and thyme essential oil, and shake well to blend.
2. Spray yourself, your clothing, and other non-food items wasps seem to be interested in.
3. Repeat this treatment as needed.

BASIL-TEA TREE WASP STING BALM

MAKES 1 TREATMENT

Wasp stings are often deep and painful. Though, unlike bees, the wasp's stinger is not left in the skin, sometimes it tears the flesh. Use this balm to stop the pain while preventing infection.

1 drop basil essential oil
1 drop tea tree essential oil

1. In a small glass bowl, add the basil and tea tree essential oils, and stir to combine.
2. Using your fingertips, apply the blend to the sting site.
3. Repeat this treatment once an hour as needed until the pain subsides.

Weight-Loss Support

Obesity complicates life in many ways. Essential oils can be used to support healthy weight loss and promote total well-being during the physical and emotional changes that accompany it.

DIFFUSE FENNEL

Not only does fennel essential oil smell terrific but it also helps promote feelings of fullness when diffused. Diffuse fennel essential oil or use it in an aromatherapy pendant. You can also add 1 or 2 drops to your bath or to a washcloth placed on the floor of your shower. Use it as often as you like to help prevent food cravings that can throw you off track.

Wrinkles

Wrinkles form as the skin loses elasticity during aging. Essential oils do not remove wrinkles; however, they can help promote healthy skin and improve elasticity, reducing the appearance of wrinkles while improving overall skin tone.

CARROT-GERANIUM TONER

MAKES 24 TREATMENTS

Carrot seed and geranium essential oils help promote elasticity and reduce the appearance of wrinkles over time.

4 ounces water
24 drops carrot seed essential oil
24 drops geranium essential oil

1. In a dark-colored glass bottle fitted with a spray top, add the water along with the carrot seed and geranium essential oils, and shake well to blend.
2. Spraying the blend generously on the face, neck, and décolletage area before moisturizing.
3. Repeat this treatment 2 times a day. Shake the bottle before each use.

ROSE-GERANIUM BEAUTY BALM

MAKES 1 TREATMENT

Rose and geranium essential oils soften the skin while promoting elasticity. This balm has a lovely fragrance that uplifts the spirit; it is sure to be a favorite.

2 drops rose essential oil
2 drops geranium essential oil

1. In a small glass bowl, add the rose and geranium essential oils, and stir to combine.
2. Using your fingertips, apply the blend to the face, neck, and décolletage area before moisturizing.
3. Repeat this treatment 1 to 3 times a day.

Yeast Infection

Yeast is a naturally occurring fungus that normally inhabits the vagina without causing problems. With a yeast infection, overgrowth causes itching, discharge, and vaginal soreness. In some cases, burning or pain is present with urination or sexual activity. Give essential oils a few days to work; if symptoms persist or worsen, contact your doctor.

TEA TREE POULTICE

MAKES 1 TREATMENT

Tea tree essential oil is a powerful antiseptic that helps stop bacteria, including yeast overgrowth, while easing the itching and discomfort that accompany a yeast infection.

1 teaspoon carrier oil
4 drops tea tree essential oil

1. In a small glass bowl, add the carrier oil and tea tree essential oil, and stir to combine.
2. Coat a tampon with the blend and insert it into the vagina, leaving it in place for 1 to 2 hours.
3. Repeat this treatment every 4 hours as needed.

MYRRH DOUCHE

MAKES 1 TREATMENT

Myrrh essential oil stops bacteria, including yeast. You can obtain a douche syringe from your local drugstore or online.

4 ounces warm water
6 drops myrrh essential oil

1. In a small glass bowl, add the water and myrrh essential oil, and stir to combine.
2. Draw the blend into a douche syringe, and use the syringe according to the manufacturer's instructions.
3. Repeat this treatment 2 times a day until the yeast infection subsides.

NATURE'S PHARMACY OF ESSENTIAL OILS

Although essential oils are used in small amounts and are usually diluted before use, they are highly concentrated and very powerful.

Dab lavender essential oil on a small burn, and watch your skin return to normal within just a few days. Use a drop of the same essential oil on your pillowcase for restful sleep, and while you're at it, rub a few drops into your pet's fur to help keep fleas away naturally. These are but a few uses for one of the world's most popular essential oils, and it is just one of the many medicinally supportive essential oils available to you in nature's abundant pharmacy.

The 75 essential oils profiled in this section are among the most popular and most versatile available. Most are surprisingly affordable, given their ability to address a wide range of ailments. Some essential oils, such as rose and neroli, are more costly. You may find it helpful to choose a few versatile essential oils to become comfortable with, then expand your collection as your confidence grows.

Although essential oils are used in small amounts and are usually diluted before use, they are highly concentrated and very powerful. Just as you wouldn't use more of a prescription drug than prescribed, don't use more of an essential oil than the recommended amount.

Allspice *Pimenta dioica*

Cooks and bakers love allspice for its ability to impart a subtly spicy note of warmth to foods sweet and savory alike. Allspice trees are native to Jamaica, though they have spread to other regions. These dense evergreens are often grown to shade coffee trees, but their real value lies in their ability to act as a natural analgesic and anesthetic. Some manufacturers market their allspice essential oil as pimento essential oil.

APPLICATION METHODS

- Use in the bath or shower for absorption and aromatherapy benefits
- Diffuse for stress, depression, and nervous tension
- Massage, diluted, for arthritis, muscle pain and stiffness, and stress

BLENDS WITH

- Bay
- Black pepper
- Camphor
- Clove
- Coriander
- Geranium
- Ginger
- Lavender
- Neroli
- Orange
- Patchouli
- Rose geranium
- Ylang-ylang

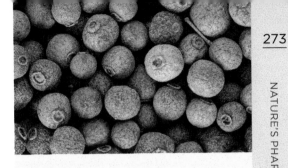

PRECAUTIONS

Allspice essential oil irritates the mucus membranes. This essential oil can be a dermal irritant for sensitive individuals. Conduct a patch test before use. Do not use neat or take internally.

- Avoid contact with mucus membranes.
- May cause skin irritation.
- Not safe for children under 6.
- Not safe for internal use.

MEDICINAL USES

Analgesic

Aphrodisiac

Arthritis

Bronchitis

Cough

Cramping

Depression

Digestive ailments

Fatigue

Flatulence

Muscle pain and stiffness

Nausea

Nervousness

Respiratory infection

Rheumatism

Stiffness

Stress

Aniseed *Pimpinella anisum*

With its sweet, licorice-like aroma, aniseed is a popular culinary staple in India and Turkey. It is also widely used in cordials and liqueurs. This beautiful annual herb grows to a maximum height of about two feet, and is prized for its delicate, feathery leaves and its tiny white flowers. Aniseed essential oil is derived from the tiny seeds produced by the flowers.

APPLICATION METHODS

- Use in the bath or shower for absorption and aromatherapy benefits
- Diffuse for asthma, cold-related problems, nausea, and vomiting
- Inhale directly for migraines and vertigo

BLENDS WITH

- Caraway
- Cardamom
- Cedarwood
- Coriander
- Dill
- Fennel
- Mandarin
- Petitgrain
- Rosewood

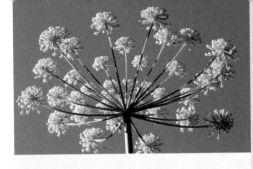

PRECAUTIONS

Aniseed essential oil is not to be confused with star anise. Aniseed essential oil solidifies at low temperatures; hand-warm the bottle before use to promote fluidity. Those with liver disease or cancer should avoid aniseed essential oil. Aniseed essential oil is phototoxic. Avoid exposing application sites to sunlight for 12 to 24 hours following application. Pregnant women should avoid aniseed essential oil.

- Avoid exposure to sunlight for 12 to 24 hours after use.
- Do not use if you are pregnant.
- Do not use if you have cancer.
- Do not use if you have liver disease.
- Do not use while breastfeeding.
- May cause skin irritation.
- Not safe for children under 6.
- Not safe for internal use.

MEDICINAL USES

Antiseptic

Anxiety

Colic

Cough

Cramping

Diuretic

Expectorant

Hangover

Indigestion

Menstrual cramps

Migraine

Muscle pain and stiffness

Nausea

Nervousness

Rheumatism

Vertigo

Whooping cough

Basil   *Ocimum basilicum*

Basil is a kitchen staple in many cultures; it grows as a perennial plant in warm climates and is cultivated as an annual favorite by gardeners in cooler climes. With a spicy-sweet, energizing fragrance, basil essential oil stimulates mind and body alike; its antibacterial and antiviral properties make it a must-have when treating ailments such as the flu or the common cold.

APPLICATION METHODS

- Use in the bath or shower for absorption and aromatherapy benefits
- Diffuse for mental alertness and migraines
- Massage, diluted, for cold, flu, and pain
- Neat on a cotton ball for earache
- Use with compress for pain

BLENDS WITH

- Bergamot
- Black pepper
- Camphor
- Caraway
- Cedarwood
- Citronella
- Clary sage
- Clove
- Fennel
- Geranium
- Ginger
- Grapefruit
- Hyssop
- Lavender
- Lemon
- Lemon eucalyptus
- Lemongrass
- Lemon verbena
- Mandarin
- Manuka
- Marjoram
- Neroli
- Orange
- Peppermint
- Rose geranium
- Rosemary
- Spearmint
- Tangerine
- Tea tree

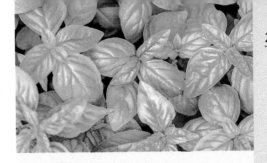

PRECAUTIONS

Basil essential oil can be a dermal irritant for sensitive individuals. Conduct a patch test before use. Those with epilepsy and cancer should avoid basil essential oil. Because it can stimulate menstrual flow, pregnant women should avoid basil essential oil.

- Do not use if you are pregnant.
- Do not use if you have cancer.
- Do not use if you have epilepsy.
- Do not use while breastfeeding.
- May cause skin irritation.
- Not safe for children under 16.
- Not safe for internal use.

MEDICINAL USES

Antibacterial	Gastric ulcers
Antiseptic	Gastric upset
Antiviral	Gout
Arthritis	Headache
Bronchitis	High
Bug bites	cholesterol
Circulatory	Mental
health	alertness
Cold	Muscle pain
Cough	and stiffness
Diabetes	Respiratory
Earache	infection
Ear infection	Rheumatism
Fatigue	Sinus infection
Flatulence	Stimulant
Flu	Tension

Bay   *Laurus nobilis*

You may use bay leaves in your kitchen, as many people around the world do. Bay trees are sturdy evergreens with long, aromatic leaves that emit a fresh, sweet, slightly spicy aroma. Bay essential oil has a similar but stronger fragrance that makes it a favorite for use in soaps, candles, and other items.

APPLICATION METHODS

- Use in the bath or shower for absorption and aromatherapy benefits
- Diffuse for emotional benefits, fever, infection, and pain
- Massage, diluted, for pain
- Use with compress for pain

BLENDS WITH

- Allspice
- Bergamot
- Cardamom
- Cedarwood
- Clary sage
- Clove
- Coriander
- Eucalyptus
- Frankincense
- Geranium
- Ginger
- Hyssop
- Juniper
- Lavender
- Lemon
- Nutmeg
- Orange
- Oregano
- Palmarosa
- Patchouli
- Pine
- Rose
- Rose geranium
- Rosemary
- Thyme
- Ylang-ylang

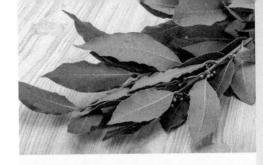

PRECAUTIONS

Bay essential oil irritates the mucus membranes. This essential oil can be a dermal irritant for sensitive individuals. Conduct a patch test before use. Those who are hemophiliacs and those taking anticoagulants should avoid bay essential oil. Those with prostate cancer, kidney disease, or liver disease should avoid this essential oil. Because it can stimulate menstrual flow, pregnant women should avoid bay essential oil.

- Avoid contact with mucus membranes.
- Do not use if you are pregnant.
- Do not use if you have cancer.
- Do not use if you have hemophilia.
- Do not use if you have kidney disease.
- Do not use if you have liver disease.
- May cause skin irritation.
- Not safe for children under 6.
- Not safe for internal use.

BASK IN PEACE, PROTECTION, AND WISDOM.

Bay essential oil was a favorite with ancient Romans, who associated it with strength, protection, wisdom, and peace. The bay tree's name is in part derived from the Latin word laudis, meaning to praise; for this reason, Olympians were presented with bay or laurel wreaths. These wreathes are symbolic of Olympic victory to this day. This useful tree has been the subject of numerous studies that have proven its antimicrobial, antifungal, and antibacterial efficacy.

MEDICINAL USES

Analgesic	Emotional
Antibacterial	balance
Antibiotic	Fever
Antifungal	Flatulence
Antimicrobial	Hair growth
Antiseptic	Healthy kidney
Bruise	function
Circulatory	Healthy liver
health	function
Cold	Infection
Creative	Neuralgia
inspiration	Oily hair
Dandruff	Psoriasis
Digestive	Rheumatism
ailments	Sprains and
Dry hair	strains
Eczema	

Benzoin   *Styrax benzoin*

Benzoin essential oil's warm, sweet aroma, which has strong notes of vanilla, makes it a staple in the perfume industry; it is also widely used in formulating incense. This essential oil is derived from the resinous sap of benzoin trees, which are native to Java, Sumatra, and Thailand.

APPLICATION METHODS

- Use in the bath or shower for absorption and aromatherapy benefits
- Diffuse for depression, emotional upset, and nervousness
- Massage, diluted, for physical ailments

BLENDS WITH

- Bergamot
- Birch
- Cedarwood
- Cinnamon
- Clove
- Coriander
- Cypress
- Fir needle
- Frankincense
- German chamomile
- Juniper
- Lavender
- Lemon
- Myrrh
- Neroli
- Orange
- Peppermint
- Petitgrain
- Roman chamomile
- Rose
- Sandalwood
- Spearmint
- Spruce

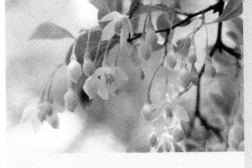

PRECAUTIONS

Benzoin essential oil has a deeply relaxing effect and should not be used prior to driving, operating machinery, or doing other tasks that require concentration.

- May act as a sedative.
- Not safe for children under 6.

MEDICINAL USES

Acne	Diabetes
Anti-inflammatory	Diuretic
	Eczema
Antiseptic	Emotional balance
Arthritis	
Bronchitis	Expectorant
Calming	Muscle pain and stiffness
Chilblains	
Circulatory health	Nervousness
	Rash
Cold	Relaxation
Cough	Scar tissue
Deodorant	Sedative
Depression	Stress

Bergamot   *Citrus bergamia*

Bergamot gets its name from the Italian city of Bergamo, which is where it was originally cultivated for use in treating digestive ailments and fevers. This delightful citrus fruit grows on trees that gain a maximum height of about 16 feet, and the essential oil is obtained from the fruit's rind. It has a fresh, spicy-sweet aroma that makes it a favorite with almost everyone who tries it, and it is widely used by fragrance manufacturers.

APPLICATION METHODS

- Use in the bath or shower for absorption and aromatherapy benefits
- Diffuse for emotional and mental benefits
- Inhale directly for emotional and mental benefits
- Massage, diluted, for physical ailments

BLENDS WITH

- Basil
- Bay
- Benzoin
- Birch
- Black pepper
- Cajeput
- Camphor
- Cardamom
- Carrot seed
- Cedarwood
- Cinnamon
- Citronella
- Clary sage
- Clover
- Coriander
- Cypress
- Fennel
- Frankincense
- Geranium
- German chamomile
- Ginger
- Grapefruit
- Helichrysum
- Jasmine
- Juniper
- Lavandin
- Lavender
- Lemon balm
- Mandarin
- Manuka
- Marjoram
- Melissa
- Myrrh
- Neroli
- Niaouli
- Nutmeg

- Orange
- Oregano
- Palmarosa
- Patchouli
- Petitgrain
- Pine
- Roman chamomile
- Rose
- Rose geranium
- Rosemary
- Rosewood
- Sandalwood
- Tagetes
- Tea tree
- Thyme
- Vetiver
- Ylang-ylang

PRECAUTIONS

Bergamot essential oil is phototoxic, so avoid exposing application sites to sunlight for 12 to 24 hours following application.

- Avoid exposure to sunlight for 12 to 24 hours after use.
- Not safe for children under 6.

MEDICINAL USES

Abscess	Infection
Acne	Itching
Analgesic	Lack of
Antibacterial	appetite
Antibiotic	Oily skin
Antiseptic	PMS
Anxiety	Psoriasis
Boil	Respiratory
Chicken pox	ailments
Cold sore	Scabies
Cystitis	Seasonal
Depression	affective
Eczema	disorder
Expectorant	Sedative
Fever	Stress
Halitosis	
Healthy liver function	

Birch *Betula alba*

Birch essential oil has a lovely balsamic fragrance that might remind you of wintergreen. Like the tree's buds, sap, twigs, and young leaflets, this essential oil is highly regarded for its usefulness in preparations for skin and hair care. It is comprised almost entirely of methyl salicylate, which is a strong pain reliever, and is an excellent essential oil to use for pain management. Birch essential oil is sometimes labeled as sweet birch, silver birch, or European white birch.

APPLICATION METHODS

- Use in the bath or shower for aromatherapy and absorption benefits
- Diffuse for aromatherapy benefits
- Massage, diluted, for physical ailments and skin care
- Use with compress for arthritis, muscle pain, and rheumatism

BLENDS WITH

- Benzoin
- Bergamot
- Grapefruit
- Jasmine
- Lemon
- Orange
- Rosemary
- Sandalwood

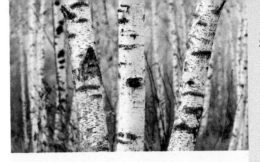

PRECAUTIONS

Birch essential oil can be a dermal irritant for sensitive individuals and should always be diluted to 25 percent or less. Those with epilepsy or who take anticoagulants should avoid birch essential oil. In addition, birch contains a high level of methyl salicylate and should not be used by those who are allergic to aspirin. Pregnant women should avoid birch essential oil.

- Do not use if you are allergic to aspirin.
- Do not use if you are pregnant.
- Do not use if you have epilepsy.
- Do not use if you take anticoagulants.
- May cause skin irritation.

MEDICINAL USES

Analgesic	Fluid retention
Antiseptic	Gout
Arthritis	Hypertension
Astringent	Insect repellent
Cellulite	Kidney stones
Circulatory health	Muscle pain
	Neuralgia
Cramping	Psoriasis
Dermatitis	Rheumatism
Disinfectant	Ringworm
Diuretic	Sciatica
Eczema	Tendinitis
Edema	Tennis elbow
Fever	Ulcers

Black Pepper   *Piper nigrum*

Fear of sneezing and eye irritation such as that which occurs with ground pepper may cause you to feel hesitant about trying black pepper essential oil. While its fragrance is similar to that of freshly ground peppercorns, it does not cause the same side effects ground pepper does. Its ability to increase stamina and alertness, paired with its value as a natural painkiller and circulatory system stimulant make it a valuable essential oil to add to your medicine chest.

APPLICATION METHODS

- Use in the bath or shower for absorption and aromatherapy benefits
- Diffuse for emotional and mental benefits
- Inhale directly for emotional and mental benefits
- Massage, diluted, for physical ailments
- Use with compress for muscle pain and stiffness

BLENDS WITH

- Allspice
- Basil
- Bergamot
- Cardamom
- Cassia
- Clary sage
- Clove
- Coriander
- Cypress
- Dill
- Fennel
- Frankincense
- Geranium
- Ginger
- Grapefruit
- Helichrysum
- Juniper
- Lavender
- Lemon
- Lemon eucalyptus
- Lemongrass
- Lime
- Mandarin
- Manuka
- Marjoram
- Nutmeg
- Orange
- Patchouli
- Peppermint
- Rosemary
- Sage
- Sandalwood
- Tangerine
- Tea tree
- Vetiver
- Ylang-ylang

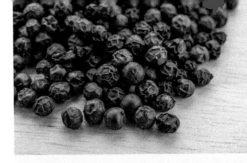

PRECAUTIONS

Black pepper essential oil can be a dermal irritant for sensitive individuals. Conduct a patch test before use. Overuse of this essential oil may cause sensitization and overstimulate the kidneys. Because it stimulates mental alertness, black pepper essential oil should not be used before sleeping. Do not combine black pepper essential oil with homeopathic remedies. Pregnant women should avoid black pepper essential oil.

- Avoid use with homeopathic remedies.
- Do not use if you are pregnant.
- May cause sensitization.
- May cause skin irritation.
- Not safe for children under 6.

MANAGE DIABETES AND HYPERTENSION NATURALLY WITH BLACK PEPPER ESSENTIAL OIL.

While you shouldn't give up necessary prescriptions, you may be able to use black pepper essential oil to help manage your health. In a 2013 study reported in the journal *Advances in Pharmacological Sciences*, key enzymes relevant to both hypertension and type 2 diabetes were positively affected by exposure to black pepper essential oil.

MEDICINAL USES

Analgesic

Antibacterial

Antiseptic

Aphrodisiac

Arthritis

Chilblains

Circulatory health

Cold

Constipation

Cramping

Diabetes

Digestive aid

Diuretic

Fatigue

Fever

Flu

Healthy kidney function

Hypertension

Laxative

Muscle pain and stiffness

Rheumatism

Cajeput   *Melaleuca leucadendra*

If you enjoy using tea tree essential oil, give cajeput a try: It's a close relative to *Melaleuca alternifolia*. With a markedly camphor-like, slightly fruity aroma, cajeput essential oil is fresh and uplifting, and it is a must-have for treating colds and flu. Also known as white tea tree and cajuput, cajeput essential oil can eliminate mental sluggishness and promote overall mental balance while easing a variety of ailments.

APPLICATION METHODS

- Use in the bath or shower for absorption and aromatherapy benefits
- Diffuse for mental stimulation and respiratory illnesses
- Massage, diluted, for physical ailments
- Use with compress for muscle pain and stiffness

BLENDS WITH

- Bergamot
- Camphor
- Clove
- Geranium
- Lavender
- Rose geranium
- Thyme

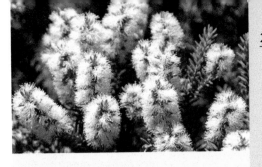

PRECAUTIONS

Cajeput essential oil can be a dermal irritant for sensitive individuals. Conduct a patch test before use.

- May cause skin irritation.
- Not safe for children under 6.

BENEFIT FROM AN ANCIENT REMEDY.
Cajeput essential oil may be one you haven't heard much about, but it has been used for millennia, both in medicine and cosmetics. Traditional remedies using cajeput include treatments for cholera, rheumatism, and stomach issues; it was and is an effective natural insecticide. This essential oil is a close relative to tea tree, and has been the subject of numerous studies that have proven its efficacy.

MEDICINAL USES

Acne

Analgesic

Antiseptic

Bronchitis

Cold

Decongestant

Digestive ailments

Earache

Expectorant

Fleas

Flu

Gout

Headache

Insecticide

Insect repellent

Intestinal parasites

Laryngitis

Lice

Menstrual support

Psoriasis

Rheumatism

Toothache

Vomiting

Calamus   *Acorus calamus var. angustatus*

Remember taking a walk through a sweetly scented woodland, and you are reminiscing about a fragrance that is close to that of calamus essential oil. Extracted from the roots of a humble wetland plant, it is an excellent oil for diffusing when experiencing emotional upset.

APPLICATION METHODS

- Use in the bath or shower for absorption and aromatherapy benefits
- Diffuse for emotional and mental benefits
- Massage, diluted, for physical ailments

BLENDS WITH

- Cedarwood
- Cinnamon
- Clary sage
- Lavender
- Patchouli
- Rosemary
- Tea tree
- Ylang-ylang

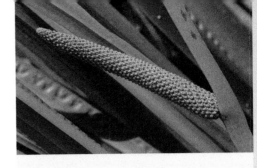

PRECAUTIONS

Do not use calamus essential oil neat or internally, as convulsions and hallucinations may result. Use a low dilution rate in massage and bath blends. Pregnant women should avoid calamus essential oil.

- Do not use if you are pregnant.
- May cause convulsions.
- Not safe for children under 6.
- Not safe for internal use.
- Not safe for neat use.

MEDICINAL USES

Anxiety

Calming

Clarity

Headache

Memory

Muscle pain and stiffness

Panic

Tension

Camphor   *Cinnamomum camphora*

When you first waft a bottle of camphor essential oil beneath your nose, you will recognize its medicinal scent immediately, as camphor is one of the active ingredients in commercially produced vapor rubs. Because this essential oil is very strong, it must be used with extreme care.

APPLICATION METHODS

- Use in the bath or shower for absorption and aromatherapy benefits
- Diffuse for aromatherapy benefits and respiratory illness
- Massage, diluted, for physical ailments
- Use with compress for muscle pain and stiffness

BLENDS WITH

- Allspice
- Basil
- Bergamot
- Cajeput
- Eucalyptus
- Frankincense
- German chamomile
- Ginger
- Lavender
- Lemon
- Melissa
- Nutmeg
- Orange
- Oregano
- Roman chamomile
- Rosemary

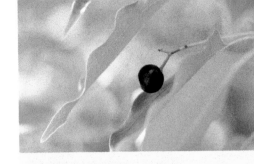

PRECAUTIONS

Overuse of camphor essential oil may cause vomiting and convulsions. Those with asthma or epilepsy should avoid camphor essential oil. Do not combine camphor essential oil with homeopathic remedies. Pregnant women should avoid camphor essential oil.

- Avoid use with homeopathic remedies.
- Do not use if you are pregnant.
- Do not use if you have asthma.
- Do not use if you have epilepsy.
- May cause convulsions.
- Not safe for children under 6.
- Not safe for internal use.

MEDICINAL USES

Acne

Analgesic

Anti-inflammatory

Antiseptic

Antiviral

Bactericidal

Bronchitis

Cold

Cough

Diuretic

Expectorant

Flu

Insecticide

Insect repellent

Intestinal parasites

Muscle pain and stiffness

Nervousness

Rheumatism

Skin care

Sprains and strains

Caraway   *Carum carvi*

Caraway is a well-known spice with a sweet, intriguing taste that makes it popular with cooks and bakers worldwide. Caraway essential oil has a slightly peppery yet sweet fragrance that makes it a pleasure to use, and its ability to effectively improve a wide range of ailments makes it a good choice for including in your medicine chest.

APPLICATION METHODS

- Use in the bath or shower for absorption and aromatherapy benefits
- Diffuse for aromatherapy benefits, digestive ailments, respiratory illness, and urinary ailments
- Massage, diluted, for physical ailments

BLENDS WITH

- Aniseed
- Basil
- Cardamom
- Cassia
- Coriander
- Dill
- Frankincense
- German chamomile
- Ginger
- Lavender
- Orange
- Roman chamomile

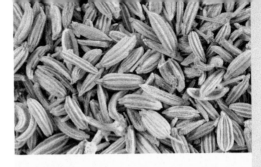

PRECAUTIONS

Caraway essential oil can be a dermal irritant for sensitive individuals. Conduct a patch test before use. Because it can stimulate menstrual flow, pregnant women should avoid caraway essential oil.

- Do not use if you are pregnant.
- May cause skin irritation.

MEDICINAL USES

Antiallergenic

Antiseptic

Asthma

Boil

Breastfeeding

Bronchitis

Colic

Cough

Disinfectant

Diuretic

Flatulence

Indigestion

Infection

Intestinal parasites

Laryngitis

Nervousness

Oily hair

Oily skin

PMS

Sore throat

Urinary ailments

Wounds

Cardamom   *Elettaria cardamomum*

If you often suffer from nausea or indigestion, consider adding cardamom essential oil to your natural apothecary. This useful oil is also an excellent remedy for coughs, edema, halitosis, and a number of other common ailments.

APPLICATION METHODS

- Use in the bath or shower for absorption and aromatherapy benefits
- Diffuse for aromatherapy benefits
- Massage, diluted, for physical ailments
- Use with compress for muscle pain and stiffness

BLENDS WITH

- Aniseed
- Bay
- Bergamot
- Black pepper
- Caraway
- Cedarwood
- Cinnamon
- Clary sage
- Clove
- Coriander
- Fennel
- Ginger
- Grapefruit
- Jasmine
- Lemon
- Lemongrass
- Mandarin
- Neroli
- Orange
- Palmarosa
- Patchouli
- Petitgrain
- Sandalwood
- Vetiver
- Ylang-ylang

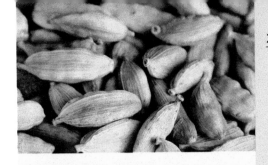

PRECAUTIONS

Cardamom essential oil is generally considered safe.

SAY GOODBYE TO BAD BREATH WITH CARDAMOM ESSENTIAL OIL. Cardamom essential oil has a far-reaching history, mentioned in ancient Ayurvedic texts as a medicinal aid for the skin and digestion. In later times, 310 BC, cardamom oil was a symbol of prosperity and royalty along with other essential oils when used in perfumes and unguents. Cardamom essential oils are not found in many perfumes today but have come full circle as an antimicrobial to treat scalp infections, skin conditions, and to promote mouth hygiene by killing germs that cause bad breath and oral thrush.

MEDICINAL USES

Antibacterial

Antiseptic

Cold

Cough

Diuretic

Edema

Expectorant

Flatulence

Halitosis

Headache

Heartburn

Laxative

Mental alertness

Nausea

Nervousness

Sciatica

Stress

Vomiting

Carrot Seed *Daucus carota*

Most people know wild carrot by its more common name: Queen Anne's lace. This flowering plant grows throughout temperate regions worldwide, and though its roots are edible, it so closely resembles poison hemlock that most foragers steer clear. Carrot seed essential oil is one of the best to have on hand for dealing with skin issues of many types as well as for detoxifying the body.

APPLICATION METHODS

- Use in the bath or shower for absorption and aromatherapy benefits
- Diffuse for aromatherapy benefits
- Massage, diluted, for physical ailments
- Use with compress for muscle pain and stiffness

BLENDS WITH

- Bergamot
- Cedarwood
- Cinnamon
- Geranium
- Ginger
- Juniper
- Lavender
- Lemon
- Lime
- Nutmeg
- Orange
- Rose geranium

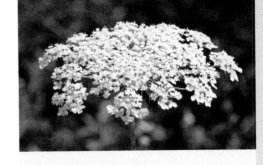

PRECAUTIONS

Because it can stimulate menstrual flow, pregnant women should avoid carrot seed essential oil.

- Do not use if you are pregnant.

COMBAT MICROORGANISMS WITH CARROT SEED ESSENTIAL OIL. Carrot seed essential oil is an excellent natural remedy to keep on hand, particularly if you want an oil that is capable of fighting fungi and bacteria. In a study reported in the December 2013 issue of *Chemistry & Biodiversity*, carrot seed essential oil was proven to exhibit antibacterial and antifungal activity against a wide range of organisms, including salmonella and E. coli.

MEDICINAL USES

Antiseptic

Arthritis

Bronchitis

Dermatitis

Detoxifier

Eczema

Edema

Fatigue

Flu

Fluid retention

Gout

Healthy liver function

Intestinal parasites

Jaundice

Muscle pain and stiffness

Rash

Rheumatism

Stimulant

Stress

Wounds

Wrinkles

Cassia   *Cinnamomum cassia*

If you enjoy curries, soft drinks, or certain baked foods or candies, it is likely that you have tasted cassia before. With a warm, pungent fragrance, this exotic essential oil comes from the leaves, branches, and bark of the cassia tree, which is a small evergreen native to China. Enjoy its uplifting fragrance and many health benefits by diffusing it in the area where you spend the most time.

APPLICATION METHODS

- Diffuse for aromatherapy benefits, colds, digestive complaints, fevers, and flu
- Massage, diluted, for arthritis and rheumatism pain

BLENDS WITH

- Black pepper
- Caraway
- Coriander
- Frankincense
- Geranium
- German chamomile
- Ginger
- Nutmeg
- Roman chamomile
- Rosemary

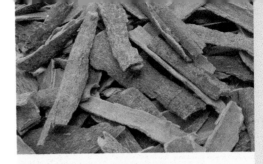

PRECAUTIONS

Cassia essential oil can be a dermal irritant for sensitive individuals. Conduct a patch test before use. Use a low dilution rate in massage and bath blends. Cassia essential oil irritates the mucus membranes.

- Avoid contact with mucus membranes.
- Do not use if you are pregnant.
- May cause skin irritation.
- Not safe for children under 6.
- Not safe for internal use.

MEDICINAL USES

Antimicrobial

Arthritis

Circulatory health

Cold

Colic

Diarrhea

Depression

Fever

Flatulence

Flu

Menstrual support

Nausea

Rheumatism

Cedarwood   *Juniperus virginiana*

Open a cedar chest or sharpen a pencil, and you'll enjoy a similar aroma to that of cedarwood essential oil. Cedar cultivars were among the first to be used for their essential oils; early Egyptians used the oil in cosmetics, as an insect repellant, and as an embalming agent. Because of its many practical and medicinal applications, cedarwood essential oil's popularity has never waned.

APPLICATION METHODS

- Use in the bath or shower for absorption and aromatherapy benefits
- Diffuse for aromatherapy benefits, arthritis, respiratory ailments, and rheumatism
- Massage, diluted, for physical ailments
- Use with compress for muscle pain and stiffness

BLENDS WITH

- Aniseed
- Basil
- Bay
- Benzoin
- Bergamot
- Calamus
- Cardamom
- Carrot seed
- Cinnamon
- Citronella
- Clary sage
- Cypress
- Eucalyptus
- Frankincense
- Ginger
- Jasmine
- Juniper
- Lavender
- Lemon
- Lemon eucalyptus
- Lemongrass
- Marjoram
- Neroli
- Oregano
- Palmarosa
- Patchouli
- Petitgrain
- Pine
- Rose
- Rose geranium
- Rosemary
- Sandalwood
- Spruce
- Valerian
- Vetiver

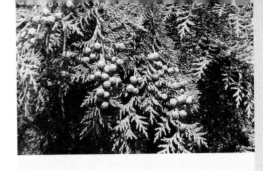

PRECAUTIONS

Cedarwood essential oil can be a dermal irritant for sensitive individuals. Conduct a patch test before use. This essential oil irritates the mucus membranes. Because it can stimulate menstrual flow, pregnant women should avoid cedarwood essential oil.

- Avoid contact with mucus membranes.
- Do not use if you are pregnant.
- May cause sensitization.
- May cause skin irritation.
- Not safe for children under 6.

MEDICINAL USES

Antiseptic

Anxiety

Arthritis

Bronchitis

Calming

Dandruff

Insect repellant

Itching

Nervousness

Oily skin

Psoriasis

Rash

Respiratory ailments

Rheumatism

Urinary tract infection

Chamomile (German) *Matricaria chamomilla, M. Recutita*

Chamomile has been used since antiquity and is among the world's most popular plants. Used to treat a wide variety of ailments, chamomile is perhaps best known for its ability to soothe and calm frayed nerves; even a single cup of tea made with the herb can help. German chamomile essential oil is closely related to Roman chamomile essential oil, and it is possible to use the two essential oils interchangeably in most cases.

APPLICATION METHODS

- Use in the bath or shower for absorption and aromatherapy benefits
- Diffuse for aromatherapy benefits
- Massage, diluted, for physical ailments
- Use neat on wounds
- Use with compress for muscle pain and stiffness

BLENDS WITH

- Benzoin
- Bergamot
- Camphor
- Caraway
- Cassia
- Clary sage
- Clove
- Cypress
- Eucalyptus
- Frankincense
- Geranium
- Grapefruit
- Helichrysum
- Jasmine
- Lavender
- Lemon
- Manuka
- Marjoram
- Melissa
- Myrrh
- Neroli
- Oregano
- Palmarosa
- Patchouli
- Rose
- Rose geranium
- Rosemary
- Tangerine
- Tea tree
- Ylang-ylang

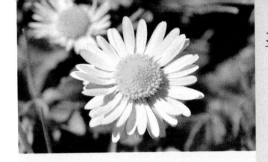

PRECAUTIONS

German chamomile essential oil has a deeply relaxing effect and should not be used prior to driving, operating machinery, or doing other tasks that require concentration. Because it can stimulate menstrual flow, pregnant women should avoid German chamomile essential oil.

- Do not use if you are pregnant.
- May act as a sedative.

MEDICINAL USES

Abscess	Headache
Acne	Insomnia
Analgesic	Measles
Anti-inflammatory	Menopausal symptoms
Anxiety	Migraine
Arthritis	Mumps
Bactericidal	Nausea
Burn	PMS
Chicken pox	Psoriasis
Cold	Sedative
Colic	Sores
Cystitis	Sprains and strains
Dental health	
Earache	Stress
Eczema	Wounds
Gingivitis	

Chamomile (Roman) *Anthemis nobilis*

If you've ever relaxed while sipping a cup of chamomile tea, you are familiar with its aroma and lightly sedative effect. Roman chamomile essential oil offers a more powerful sedative property than does German chamomile, and its fragrance is a bit sweeter. If you are selecting just a few essential oils to keep on hand, consider making this one of them. Its anti-inflammatory action is impressive, and its usefulness in addressing skin complaints, headaches, and stress-related conditions is remarkable.

APPLICATION METHODS

- Use in the bath or shower for absorption and aromatherapy benefits
- Diffuse for aromatherapy benefits
- Gargle, diluted, for tonsillitis
- Massage, diluted, for physical ailments
- Use as mouthwash for dental health
- Use neat on wounds
- Use with compress for muscle pain and stiffness

BLENDS WITH

- Bergamot
- Camphor
- Caraway
- Cassia
- Clary sage
- Clove
- Cypress
- Eucalyptus
- Geranium
- Grapefruit
- Jasmine
- Lavender
- Lemon
- Mandarin
- Manuka
- Melissa
- Myrrh
- Neroli
- Oakmoss
- Oregano
- Palmarosa
- Patchouli
- Rose
- Rose geranium
- Tangerine
- Tea tree
- Ylang-ylang

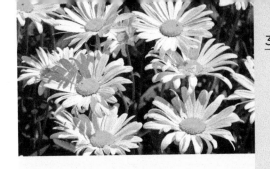

PRECAUTIONS

Roman chamomile essential oil has a deeply relaxing effect and should not be used prior to driving, operating machinery, or doing other tasks that require concentration. Because it can stimulate menstrual flow, pregnant women should avoid Roman chamomile essential oil.

- Do not use if you are pregnant.
- May act as a sedative.

MEDICINAL USES

Abscess	Diaper rash
Acne	Earache
Addiction	Eczema
Analgesic	Gingivitis
Anger	Headache
Antiallergenic	Insomnia
Anti-inflammatory	Irritability
	Migraine
Anxiety	Nausea
Arthritis	Psoriasis
Bactericidal	Sedative
Boil	Sores
Burn	Sprains and strains
Chicken pox	
Cold	Sunburn
Colic	Stress
Cystitis	Tonsillitis
Dental health	Wounds

Cinnamon   *Cinnamomum zeylanicum, C. verum*

When most people think of cinnamon, visions of delicious baked goods are often the first thing to come to mind. Besides its value in culinary applications, cinnamon offers superb benefits when used in natural medicines. Cinnamon essential oil has a spicy, somewhat musky fragrance that may remind you more of incense than anything else.

APPLICATION METHODS

- Use in the bath or shower for absorption and aromatherapy benefits
- Diffuse for aromatherapy benefits and respiratory ailments
- Massage, diluted, for physical ailments

BLENDS WITH

- Benzoin
- Bergamot
- Calamus
- Cardamom
- Carrot seed
- Cedarwood
- Clove
- Coriander
- Dill
- Elemi
- Frankincense
- Ginger
- Grapefruit
- Lavandin
- Lavender
- Lemon
- Mandarin
- Marjoram
- Nutmeg
- Orange
- Patchouli
- Peppermint
- Petitgrain
- Rose
- Rosemary
- Tangerine
- Thyme
- Ylang-ylang

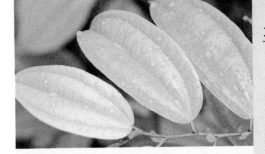

PRECAUTIONS

Make sure that you choose cinnamon essential oil extracted from the leaves, rather than the bark of the cinnamon tree. Cinnamon bark essential oil is of little use in aromatherapy and is a strong dermal toxin. Cinnamon leaf essential oil should be used with care. Because it can stimulate menstrual flow, pregnant women should avoid cinnamon essential oil. Those with hemophilia, prostate cancer, kidney disease or liver disease should avoid cinnamon essential oil. Those taking anticoagulants should avoid cinnamon essential oil. It can be a dermal irritant for sensitive individuals. Conduct a patch test before use. Cinnamon essential oil irritates the mucus membranes.

- Avoid contact with mucus membranes.
- Do not use if you are pregnant.
- Do not use if you have hemophilia.
- Do not use if you have kidney disease.
- Do not use if you have liver disease.
- Do not use if you have prostate cancer.
- May cause skin irritation.
- Not safe for children under 6.
- Not safe for internal use.

MEDICINAL USES

Analgesic

Antibacterial

Antibiotic

Antiseptic

Aphrodisiac

Arthritis

Bronchitis

Cold

Depression

Diarrhea

Disinfectant

Fever

Insecticide

Intestinal parasites

Menstrual support

Respiratory infection

Rheumatism

Citronella   *Cymbopogon nardus, Andropogon nardus*

Popularized for its usefulness in repelling mosquitoes and other bothersome bugs, citronella essential oil is useful for a number of applications. Extracted from tall grass native to Java and Sri Lanka, it has a lightly sweet citrus aroma. Ensure you purchase citronella essential oil rather than something labeled as *citronella oil*. The latter usually has a paraffin or mineral oil base and is typically meant for use as an outdoor insect repellent.

APPLICATION METHODS

- Use in the bath or shower for absorption and aromatherapy benefits
- Diffuse for aromatherapy benefits and as an insect repellent
- Massage, diluted, for physical ailments
- Spray for insect repellent on body, clothing, and other items

BLENDS WITH

- Basil
- Bergamot
- Cedarwood
- Geranium
- Lavandin
- Lavender
- Lemon
- Lime
- Orange
- Oregano
- Pine
- Rose geranium
- Rosemary
- Sandalwood

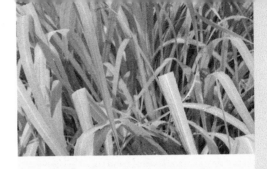

PRECAUTIONS

Citronella essential oil may cause sensitization and irritate mucus membranes. Those with an estrogen-dependent cancer should avoid citronella essential oil. Because it can stimulate menstrual flow, pregnant women should avoid citronella essential oil.

- Avoid contact with mucus membranes.
- Do not use if you are pregnant.
- Do not use if you have an estrogen-dependent cancer.
- May cause sensitization.
- Not safe for children under 6.

MEDICINAL USES

Analgesic

Antibacterial

Antifungal

Antiseptic

Cold

Fatigue

Fever

Fleas

Flu

Foot odor

Headache

Indoor air freshener

Insecticide

Insect repellent

Intestinal parasites

Oily skin

Clary Sage *Salvia sclarea*

While common garden sage is well known for its ability to add flavor to savory dishes, clary sage is best known for its medicinal value. Clary sage essential oil is one of the most important essential oils to keep on hand for menstrual complaints, menopausal symptoms, and treating minor wounds. Its pleasant, nutty fragrance can bring relaxation even during periods of intense stress.

APPLICATION METHODS

- Use in the bath or shower for absorption and aromatherapy benefits
- Diffuse for aromatherapy benefits
- Massage, diluted, for physical ailments
- Use with compress for muscle pain and stiffness

BLENDS WITH

- Basil
- Bay
- Bergamot
- Black pepper
- Calamus
- Cardamom
- Cedarwood
- Clove
- Coriander
- Cypress
- Frankincense
- Geranium
- German chamomile
- Grapefruit
- Helichrysum
- Hyssop
- Jasmine
- Juniper
- Lavandin
- Lavender
- Lemon balm
- Lemon eucalyptus
- Lemongrass
- Lime
- Mandarin
- Manuka
- Neroli
- Nutmeg
- Orange
- Palmarosa
- Patchouli
- Petitgrain
- Pine
- Roman chamomile
- Rose
- Rose geranium
- Rosemary
- Sandalwood
- Spikenard
- Spruce
- Tagetes
- Tea tree
- Vetiver
- Ylang-ylang

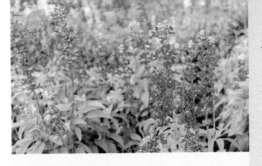

PRECAUTIONS

Clary sage essential oil has a deeply relaxing effect and should not be used prior to driving, operating machinery, or doing other tasks that require concentration. Do not use it with alcohol or sedatives. Overuse of clary sage essential oil can cause headaches. Because it can stimulate menstrual flow, pregnant women should avoid clary sage essential oil.

- Do not use if you are pregnant.
- May act as a sedative.
- May cause sensitization.
- Not safe for children under 6.

MEDICINAL USES

Acne

Antibacterial

Antifungal

Anti-inflammatory

Antiseptic

Aphrodisiac

Boil

Calming

Childbirth support

Depression

Digestive ailments

Emotional balance

Flatulence

Insomnia

Irritability

Joint pain

Kidney disease

Menopause support

Menstrual support

Muscle pain and stiffness

PMS

Rash

Sedative

Sore throat

Stress

Wounds

Clove *Syzygium aromaticum, Eugenia caryophyllata*

Highly aromatic and prized for their ability to impart sweet, spicy flavor to foods, cloves have been used for their medicinal qualities throughout history. Like ancient Chinese, Greek, and Roman people who used clove to sweeten their breath and ease toothaches, you can take advantage of this essential oil's ability to ease dental woes. Its ability to relieve pain, speed healing, and ease respiratory problems are just a few more reasons to make this one of the essential oils you keep on hand for regular use.

APPLICATION METHODS

- Use in the bath or shower for absorption and aromatherapy benefits
- Diffuse for aromatherapy benefits
- Massage, diluted, for physical ailments
- Use with compress for muscle pain and stiffness

BLENDS WITH

- Allspice
- Basil
- Bay
- Benzoin
- Bergamot
- Black pepper
- Cajeput
- Cardamom
- Cinnamon
- Clary sage
- Coriander
- Geranium
- German chamomile
- Ginger
- Grapefruit
- Helichrysum
- Jasmine
- Lavender
- Lemon
- Lemon eucalyptus
- Mandarin
- Myrrh
- Orange
- Palmarosa
- Patchouli
- Petitgrain
- Roman chamomile
- Rose
- Rose geranium
- Sandalwood
- Spikenard
- Tangerine
- Tea tree
- Ylang-ylang

PRECAUTIONS

Clove essential oil can be a dermal irritant for sensitive individuals. Conduct a patch test before use. This essential oil irritates the mucus membranes. Those with cancer should avoid clove essential oil. Do not use clove essential oil during pregnancy.

- Do not use if you are pregnant.
- Do not use if you have cancer.
- May cause skin irritation.
- Not safe for children under 6.
- Not safe for internal use.

CLOVE ESSENTIAL OIL IS A POWERFUL INSECTICIDE. In a 2010 study reported by the medical journal *PLOS ONE*, clove essential oil was shown to be effective against scabies mites. Nutmeg and ylang-ylang essential oils were studied during the same testing period, with nutmeg showing some efficacy against the mites and ylang-ylang showing very little.

MEDICINAL USES

Aging skin

Analgesic

Antibacterial

Antifungal

Anti-inflammatory

Antimicrobial

Antiseptic

Antiviral

Asthma

Bronchitis

Dental health

Diarrhea

Expectorant

Insecticide

Insect repellant

Intestinal parasites

Muscle pain and stiffness

Rheumatism

Scabies

Skin problems

Toothache

Vomiting

Coriander *Coriandrum sativum*

Coriander's famous flavor has made its way into liqueurs such as Benedictine and Chartreuse. The plant's seeds, which were used as an aphrodisiac by Egyptians, were found in King Tutankhamun's tomb. Coriander essential oil's aroma is sweet, herbaceous, and slightly spicy, and like many foods containing the herb, it is useful for calming the digestive system. Use it for detoxification, migraine relief, muscle spasms, and more.

APPLICATION METHODS

- Use in the bath or shower for absorption and aromatherapy benefits
- Diffuse for aromatherapy benefits and to stimulate appetite
- Massage, diluted, for physical ailments

BLENDS WITH

- Allspice
- Aniseed
- Bay
- Benzoin
- Bergamot
- Black pepper
- Caraway
- Cardamom
- Cassia
- Cinnamon
- Clary sage
- Clove
- Cypress
- Frankincense
- Geranium
- Ginger
- Grapefruit
- Jasmine
- Lemon
- Lemongrass
- Neroli
- Nutmeg
- Orange
- Palmarosa
- Patchouli
- Petitgrain
- Ravensara
- Sandalwood
- Vetiver
- Ylang-ylang

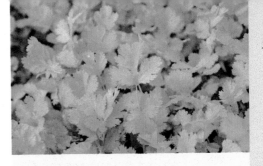

PRECAUTIONS

Coriander essential oil can be a dermal irritant for sensitive individuals. Conduct a patch test before use. Overuse of this essential oil may cause stupor.

- May cause skin irritation.
- May cause stupor.

TREAT IRRITABLE BOWEL SYNDROME NATURALLY WITH CORIANDER. Coriander essential oil has been proven effective against E. coli, bacteria which often play a role in irritable bowel syndrome. In a study reported by the journal *BMC Complementary and Alternative Medicine*, coriander essential oil was shown to be more effective than the antibiotic rifaximin in combating E. coli. Peppermint and lemon balm essential oils were also proven effective, with peppermint showing greater efficacy than lemon balm.

MEDICINAL USES

Analgesic

Antibacterial

Aphrodisiac

Arthritis

Colic

Cramping

Fatigue

Flatulence

Fungicidal

Indigestion

Migraine

Muscle pain and stiffness

Nausea

Rheumatism

Stress

Cypress *Cupressus sempervirens*

With its refreshing, evergreen aroma and its ability to soothe stress, ease tension, and mitigate anger and irritability, cypress essential oil is an excellent choice for your home apothecary. Its ability to promote healing, improve circulation, and relieve cold and flu symptoms makes it even more valuable.

APPLICATION METHODS

- Use in the bath or shower for absorption and aromatherapy benefits
- Diffuse for aromatherapy benefits
- Massage, diluted, for physical ailments
- Use with compress for muscle pain and stiffness
- Use with ice pack for nosebleeds

BLENDS WITH

- Benzoin
- Bergamot
- Black pepper
- Cedarwood
- Clary sage
- Coriander
- Eucalyptus
- Fennel
- Frankincense
- Geranium
- German chamomile
- Ginger
- Grapefruit
- Helichrysum
- Juniper
- Lavender
- Lemon eucalyptus
- Lemongrass
- Manuka
- Marjoram
- Myrrh
- Oregano
- Peppermint
- Petitgrain
- Pine
- Roman chamomile
- Rose geranium
- Spikenard
- Tea tree
- Ylang-ylang

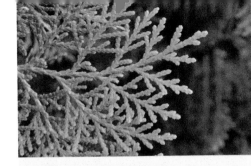

PRECAUTIONS

■ Do not use if you are pregnant.

**CLEAR YOUR MIND AND GAIN COMFORT FROM
CYPRESS.** Cypress trees were worshiped as a symbol
of Beruth, the Earth goddess, on the island of Cyprus,
and were thought to encourage contemplation in
China because the roots of the tree look like a seated
figure. Similar to this rich history, cypress essential
oil is thought to clear and soothe the mind. Cypress
trees are forever linked through literature and art
with mourning, death, and eternal rest. This is why
cypress wood is still used today for coffins and
these evergreens are planted in cemeteries in the
United States.

MEDICINAL USES

Anger	Hemorrhoids
Antibacterial	Insecticide
Anti-inflammatory	Insect repellant
	Irritability
Antiseptic	Menstrual
Bronchitis	support
Calming	Nosebleed
Cold	PMS
Cough	Sedative
Diaper rash	Stress
Diuretic	Styptic
Emphysema	Varicose veins
Expectorant	Whooping
Fever	cough
Foot odor	

Dill   *Anethum graveolens*

People love dill for its enticing aroma and clean, refreshing flavor. Essential oil made from the herb has some of the same characteristics, with a pleasing, earthy undertone. Its soothing properties affect body and mind alike, making it an excellent oil to keep on hand.

APPLICATION METHODS

- Use in the bath or shower for absorption and aromatherapy benefits
- Diffuse for aromatherapy benefits
- Massage, diluted, for physical ailments
- Use with compress for muscle pain and stiffness

BLENDS WITH

- Aniseed
- Black pepper
- Caraway
- Cinnamon
- Clove
- Elemi
- Fennel
- Lemon
- Lime
- Nutmeg
- Orange
- Peppermint
- Spearmint

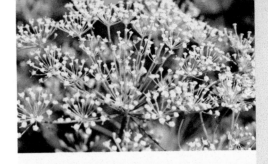

PRECAUTIONS

Do not use dill essential oil during pregnancy. Dill essential oil is phototoxic. Avoid exposing application sites to sunlight for 12 to 24 hours following application.

- Do not use if you are pregnant.
- Avoid exposure to sunlight for 12 to 24 hours after use.

MEDICINAL USES

Bactericidal

Breastfeeding

Constipation

Disinfectant

Flatulence

Hiccups

Indigestion

Menstrual cramps

Nervousness

Sedative

Wounds

Elemi   *Canarium luzonicum*

If you enjoy using frankincense or myrrh essential oils, you are very likely to appreciate elemi essential oil. Like its close relatives, it is sourced from tree resin and is useful for improving skin tone and texture, promoting wound healing, and soothing muscles and mind alike.

APPLICATION METHODS

- Use in the bath or shower for absorption and aromatherapy benefits
- Diffuse for aromatherapy benefits and respiratory ailments
- Massage, diluted, for physical ailments
- Neat for muscle pain, scarring, and stiffness

BLENDS WITH

- Cinnamon
- Dill
- Frankincense
- Juniper
- Lavender
- Lemon verbena
- Myrrh
- Rosemary
- Sage

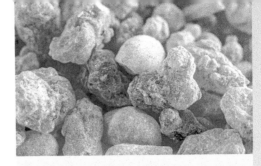

PRECAUTIONS

Elemi essential oil can be a dermal irritant for sensitive individuals. Conduct a patch test before use.

- May cause skin irritation.

MEDICINAL USES

Aging skin

Analgesic

Antiseptic

Antiviral

Bronchitis

Cough

Emotional balance

Expectorant

Fungicidal

Muscle pain and stiffness

Nervousness

Relaxation

Scarring

Skin infection

Stress

Wounds

Eucalyptus *Eucalyptus globulus, E. radiata*

Many people find the fresh, clean scent of eucalyptus essential oil irresistible, but its uplifting fragrance isn't the only reason to keep it on hand. Eucalyptus essential oil is a key ingredient in nontoxic household cleaners, a go-to remedy for colds and the flu, a wonderful treatment for sore muscles, and much more.

APPLICATION METHODS

- Use in the bath or shower for absorption and aromatherapy benefits
- Diffuse for aromatherapy benefits
- Massage, diluted, for physical ailments
- Use with compress for muscle pain and stiffness

BLENDS WITH

- Bay
- Camphor
- Cedarwood
- Cypress
- Geranium
- German chamomile
- Ginger
- Grapefruit
- Juniper
- Lavender
- Lemon
- Lemon eucalyptus
- Manuka
- Marjoram
- Niaouli
- Orange
- Oregano
- Peppermint
- Petitgrain
- Pine
- Roman chamomile
- Rosemary
- Spearmint
- Tea tree
- Thyme

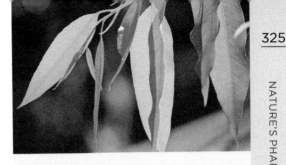

PRECAUTIONS

Do not use eucalyptus essential oil internally. Do not combine eucalyptus essential oil with homeopathic remedies. Those with an estrogen-dependent cancer should avoid eucalyptus essential oil.

- Avoid use with homeopathic remedies.
- Do not use if you are pregnant.
- Do not use if you have an estrogen-dependent cancer.
- Not safe for children under 6.
- Not safe for internal use.

EASE BRONCHITIS SYMPTOMS WITH EUCALYPTUS ESSENTIAL OIL. This powerful essential oil contains monoterpenes, which are effective in treating respiratory illnesses; in fact, in one study published in the international journal *Arzneimittelforschung* now known as *Drug Research*, bronchitis sufferers who used eucalyptus essential oil did as well as those study participants who were given antibiotics.

MEDICINAL USES

Acne

Analgesic

Antibacterial

Antifungal

Antiseptic

Antiviral

Arthritis

Bronchitis

Candida

Cold

Cough

Decongestant

Diuretic

Expectorant

Fever

Flu

Intestinal parasites

Migraine

Muscle pain and stiffness

Rheumatism

Sinus infection

Fennel   *Foeniculum vulgare*

The popularity of fennel dates back to ancient Romans and Egyptians, who used the licorice-scented herb medicinally for such ailments as earaches and snake bites, and spiritually to impart longevity, courage, and strength. Fennel is a favorite essential oil today for its ability to minimize hunger, ease digestive problems, stimulate estrogen production, and more.

APPLICATION METHODS

- Use in the bath or shower for absorption and aromatherapy benefits
- Diffuse for aromatherapy benefits
- Massage, diluted, for physical ailments
- Neat on inflammation and for pain relief
- Use with compress for muscle pain and stiffness

BLENDS WITH

- Aniseed
- Basil
- Bergamot
- Black pepper
- Cardamom
- Cypress
- Dill
- Geranium
- Ginger
- Grapefruit
- Juniper
- Lavender
- Lemon
- Lemongrass
- Mandarin
- Marjoram
- Melissa
- Niaouli
- Orange
- Pine
- Ravensara
- Rose
- Rose geranium
- Rosemary
- Sandalwood
- Tangerine
- Ylang-ylang

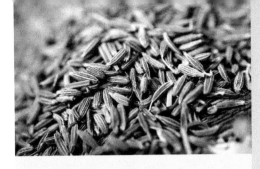

PRECAUTIONS

Those with epilepsy or cancer should avoid fennel essential oil. Because it can stimulate menstrual flow, pregnant women should avoid fennel essential oil.

- Do not use if you are pregnant.
- Do not use if you have epilepsy.
- Do not use if you have cancer.
- Not safe for children under 6.
- Not safe for internal use.

MEDICINAL USES

Analgesic

Antibacterial

Antifungal

Anti-inflammatory

Antimicrobial

Antiseptic

Childbirth

Diabetes

Diuretic

Estrogen production

Fluid retention

Intestinal parasites

Kidney stones

Menstrual support

Perimenopause

PMS

Urinary tract infection

Weight-loss support

Fir Needle *Abies balsamea, A. alba*

If walking in an evergreen forest on a warm day stirs your senses, you are certain to enjoy fir needle essential oil. For many, its fragrance is reminiscent of a fresh-cut Christmas tree—woody, sweet, balsamic, and a little earthy. This useful essential oil is ideal for imparting indoor air with an uplifting fragrance while killing airborne germs. It is prized for its ability to ease muscle pain and stiffness, arthritis, rheumatism, and other body pain.

APPLICATION METHODS

- Use in the bath or shower for absorption and aromatherapy benefits
- Diffuse for aromatherapy benefits
- Massage, diluted, for physical ailments
- Use with compress for muscle pain and stiffness

BLENDS WITH

- Benzoin
- Lavender
- Lemon
- Marjoram
- Orange
- Pine
- Rosemary

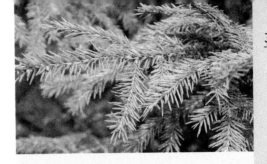

PRECAUTIONS

Fir needle essential oil can be a dermal irritant for sensitive individuals. Conduct a patch test before use.

- May cause skin irritation.

MEDICINAL USES

Analgesic

Antimicrobial

Antiseptic

Arthritis

Bronchitis

Cold

Cough

Expectorant

Flu

Muscle pain and stiffness

Rheumatism

Sinus infection

Frankincense   *Boswellia carteri*

Early Sumerians and Egyptians used frankincense essential oil for incense, stomach ailments, skin care, and cosmetics; today, it continues to be prized for its usefulness. The aroma of frankincense stimulates the brain's emotional center, soothing and calming the mind. Physically, frankincense essential oil strengthens the immune system, aids in rejuvenating skin and promoting healing, and helps compromised respiratory systems recover. If you are looking for an essential oil with the ability to improve mind and body alike, consider frankincense.

APPLICATION METHODS

- Use in the bath or shower for absorption and aromatherapy benefits
- Diffuse for aromatherapy benefits and respiratory ailments
- Massage, diluted, for physical ailments
- Use with compress for muscle pain and stiffness

BLENDS WITH

- Bay
- Benzoin
- Bergamot
- Black pepper
- Camphor
- Caraway
- Cassia
- Cedarwood
- Cinnamon
- Clary sage
- Coriander
- Cypress
- Elemi
- Geranium
- German chamomile
- Ginger
- Grapefruit
- Lavender
- Lemon
- Lemon eucalyptus
- Mandarin
- Myrrh
- Neroli
- Orange
- Palmarosa
- Patchouli
- Petitgrain
- Pine
- Rose
- Rose geranium
- Rosemary
- Sandalwood
- Spikenard
- Vetiver
- Ylang-ylang

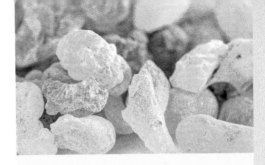

PRECAUTIONS

Because it can stimulate menstrual flow, pregnant women should avoid frankincense essential oil.

- Do not use if you are pregnant.

MEDICINAL USES

Aging skin
Analgesic
Antifungal
Anti-
   inflammatory
Antiseptic
Anxiety
Asthma
Bedsores
Bronchitis
Carbuncles
Cold
Cough
Diaper rash
Diuretic

Emotional
   balance
Expectorant
Fatigue
Flu
Laryngitis
Menstrual
   support
Nightmares
Rheumatism
Scars
Sedative
Stretch marks
Wounds

Geranium   *Pelargonium odorantissimum*

People appreciate geraniums for their vivid blooms and delightful herbaceous fragrance. Geranium essential oil has a beautiful floral aroma with an underlying hint of mint. Traditionally used to balance the emotions and hormones, stimulate the lymph system, and to help a variety of skin conditions, it is also useful as a natural insect repellent and insecticide.

APPLICATION METHODS

- Use in the bath or shower for absorption and aromatherapy benefits
- Diffuse for aromatherapy benefits
- Massage, diluted, for physical ailments
- Neat for wrinkled skin and wounds
- Use with compress for muscle pain and stiffness

BLENDS WITH

- Allspice
- Basil
- Bay
- Bergamot
- Black pepper
- Cajeput
- Carrot seed
- Cassia
- Citronella
- Clary sage
- Clove
- Coriander
- Cypress
- Eucalyptus
- Fennel
- Frankincense
- German chamomile
- Ginger
- Grapefruit
- Helichrysum
- Hyssop
- Jasmine
- Juniper
- Lavender
- Lemon
- Lemon eucalyptus
- Lemongrass
- Mandarin
- Manuka
- Melissa
- Myrrh
- Neroli
- Nutmeg
- Orange
- Palmarosa
- Patchouli

- Peppermint
- Petitgrain
- Roman chamomile
- Rose
- Rose geranium
- Rosemary
- Rosewood
- Sandalwood
- Spikenard
- Tangerine
- Tea tree
- Vetiver
- Ylang-ylang

PRECAUTIONS

Geranium essential oil can be a dermal irritant for sensitive individuals. Conduct a patch test before use. Geranium essential oil has a deeply relaxing effect and should not be used prior to driving, operating machinery, or doing other tasks that require concentration. Because it can stimulate menstrual flow, pregnant women should avoid geranium essential oil.

- Do not use if you are pregnant.
- May act as a sedative.
- May cause skin irritation.
- Not safe for children under 6.

MEDICINAL USES

Acne	Lice
Aging skin	Menopause
Analgesic	support
Antibacterial	PMS
Antiseptic	Ringworm
Anxiety	Sedative
Bruise	Shingles
Burn	Skin care
Cellulite	Sore throat
Circulatory	Stress
health	Styptic
Depression	Tonsillitis
Diuretic	Vasoconstrictor
Insecticide	Wounds
Insect repellant	
Intestinal	
parasites	

Ginger *Zingiber officinale*

Ginger's sweet, spicy taste makes it a favorite with chefs and bakers everywhere, and its use in herbal medicine is far-reaching. Ginger essential oil offers the concentrated power of ginger, soothing a wide range of digestive maladies, offering relief from pain, and helping alleviate cold and flu symptoms.

APPLICATION METHODS

- Use in the bath or shower for absorption and aromatherapy benefits
- Diffuse for aromatherapy benefits
- Massage, diluted, for physical ailments
- Use with compress for muscle pain and stiffness

BLENDS WITH

- Allspice
- Basil
- Bay
- Bergamot
- Black pepper
- Camphor
- Caraway
- Cardamom
- Cassia
- Cedarwood
- Cinnamon
- Clove
- Coriander
- Cypress
- Eucalyptus
- Fennel
- Frankincense
- Geranium
- Grapefruit
- Jasmine
- Juniper
- Lemon
- Lemon eucalyptus
- Lemongrass
- Lime
- Mandarin
- Neroli
- Orange
- Palmarosa
- Patchouli
- Rose
- Rose geranium
- Sandalwood
- Vetiver
- Ylang-ylang

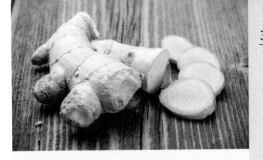

PRECAUTIONS

Ginger essential oil can be a dermal irritant for sensitive individuals. Conduct a patch test before use. It is also phototoxic. Avoid exposing application sites to sunlight for 12 to 24 hours following application. Because it can stimulate menstrual flow, pregnant women should avoid ginger essential oil.

- Avoid exposure to sunlight for 12 to 24 hours after use.
- Do not use if you are pregnant.
- May cause skin irritation.

MEDICINAL USES

Analgesic	Expectorant
Antibacterial	Fever
Anti-inflammatory	Flu
Antiseptic	Laxative
Aphrodisiac	Libido
Arthritis	Morning sickness
Circulatory health	Motion sickness
Cold	Muscle pain and stiffness
Cough	Nausea
Cramping	Seasonal affective disorder
Decongestant	
Depression	
Diarrhea	
Diuretic	

Grapefruit *Citrus paradisi*

Grapefruit is a refreshing addition to breakfast, and many people find that the scent of the freshly peeled fruit uplifts their spirits. Grapefruit essential oil has an even more powerful effect, stimulating the mind and promoting feelings of happiness. It is often used as a diuretic; however, its usefulness extends to skin and hair care, antiseptic applications, and much more.

APPLICATION METHODS

- Use in the bath or shower for absorption and aromatherapy benefits
- Diffuse for aromatherapy benefits
- Massage, diluted, for physical ailments
- Use with compress for muscle pain and stiffness

BLENDS WITH

- Basil
- Bergamot
- Birch
- Black pepper
- Cardamom
- Cinnamon
- Clary sage
- Clove
- Coriander
- Cypress
- Eucalyptus
- Fennel
- Frankincense
- Geranium
- German chamomile
- Ginger
- Hyssop
- Juniper
- Lavender
- Lemon
- Lemongrass
- Mandarin
- Manuka
- Myrrh
- Neroli
- Orange
- Palmarosa
- Patchouli
- Peppermint
- Pine
- Roman chamomile
- Rose geranium
- Rosemary
- Tangerine
- Thyme
- Vetiver
- Ylang-ylang

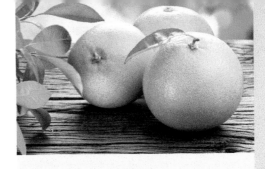

PRECAUTIONS

Grapefruit essential oil can be a dermal irritant for sensitive individuals. Conduct a patch test before use. It is also phototoxic. Avoid exposing application sites to sunlight for 12 to 24 hours following application.

- Avoid exposure to sunlight for 12 to 24 hours after use.
- May cause skin irritation.

MEDICINAL USES

Acne

Antibacterial

Antiseptic

Cellulite

Depression

Detoxification

Diuretic

Fatigue

Hangover

Headache

Irritability

Lymph stimulant

Muscle pain and stiffness

Oily hair

Oily skin

Weight-loss support

Helichrysum *Helichrysum italicum*

Many people find helichrysum's honey-like fragrance to be cloyingly sweet, but this oil is used more for physical healing than for aromatherapy applications. Its regenerative quality makes it ideal for treating a wide range of injuries and skin conditions, including more severe issues such as sprains and hematomas.

APPLICATION METHODS

- Use in the bath or shower for absorption and aromatherapy benefits
- Diffuse for aromatherapy benefits
- Massage, diluted, for physical ailments
- Neat for compromised skin and stretch marks
- Use with compress for muscle pain and stiffness

BLENDS WITH

- Bergamot
- Black pepper
- Clary sage
- Clove
- Cypress
- Geranium
- German chamomile
- Juniper
- Lavender
- Lemon
- Neroli
- Orange
- Palmarosa
- Rosemary
- Tea tree
- Thyme
- Vetiver
- Ylang-ylang

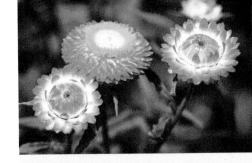

PRECAUTIONS

Helichrysum essential oil is generally considered safe.

FADE YOUR SCARS AND STRETCH MARKS WITH HELICHRYSUM. Helichrysum essential oil has a long history stretching back to ancient times when it was used to unlock the possibilities of a spiritual existence by uncluttering the mind. Over the years, the use of this essential oil has evolved to eliminating scars of a physical nature rather than soothing spiritual ones. The University of Nigeria conducted a study that showed that rubbing helichrysum essential oil on stretch marks and scars, even old ones, could fade them significantly.

MEDICINAL USES

Abscess

Acne

Aging skin

Antiallergenic

Antibacterial

Anti-inflammatory

Antimicrobial

Boil

Bruise

Burn

Dermatitis

Diuretic

Eczema

Expectorant

Rash

Scars

Sprains and strains

Stretch marks

Wounds

Hyssop *Hyssopus officinalis*

Hyssop is a fragrant herb that was used by Romans for purification; it is mentioned in the Bible for its ability to soothe chest ailments and the effects of leprosy. In the past, the herb was used to ward off lice, flavor liqueur, and feed honeybees; today, hyssop essential oil continues to offer solutions to a wide range of physical ailments and emotional woes.

APPLICATION METHODS

- Use in the bath or shower for absorption and aromatherapy benefits
- Diffuse for aromatherapy benefits
- Massage, diluted, for physical ailments
- Use with compress for muscle pain and stiffness

BLENDS WITH

- Basil
- Bay
- Clary sage
- Geranium
- Grapefruit
- Lavender
- Lemon
- Mandarin
- Myrtle
- Orange
- Rosemary
- Sage

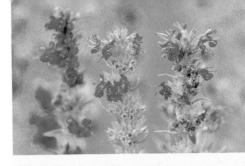

PRECAUTIONS

Those with epilepsy should avoid hyssop essential oil. Do not use hyssop essential oil internally. Because it can stimulate menstrual flow, pregnant women should avoid hyssop essential oil.

- Do not use if you are pregnant.
- Do not use if you have epilepsy.
- Not safe for children under 12.
- Not safe for internal use.

MEDICINAL USES

Antibacterial

Anti-inflammatory

Antiseptic

Antiviral

Anxiety

Bronchitis

Bruise

Cold

Cough

Dermatitis

Diuretic

Eczema

Emotional balance

Expectorant

Fatigue

Fever

Flu

Intestinal parasites

Lice

Mental alertness

Wounds

Jasmine   *Jasminum officinale*

The sweet smell of jasmine is unmistakable—and unforgettable. A favorite with many, jasmine essential oil has the ability to alleviate depression, ease respiratory illness, mitigate menstrual problems, and perform a number of other useful functions. While this is one of the more costly essential oils available, its usefulness outweighs its price tag.

APPLICATION METHODS

- Use in the bath or shower for absorption and aromatherapy benefits
- Diffuse for aromatherapy benefits
- Inhale directly for addiction, depression, and stress
- Massage, diluted, for physical ailments
- Neat for dry skin, muscle pain and stiffness, scarring, and stretch marks
- Use with compress for muscle pain and stiffness

BLENDS WITH

- Bergamot
- Birch
- Cardamom
- Cedarwood
- Clary sage
- Clove
- Coriander
- Geranium
- German chamomile
- Ginger
- Lavandin
- Lemon
- Lime
- Mandarin
- Myrrh
- Neroli
- Orange
- Patchouli
- Petitgrain
- Roman chamomile
- Rose
- Rose geranium
- Rosewood
- Sandalwood
- Spearmint
- Tagetes
- Tangerine
- Vetiver
- Ylang-ylang

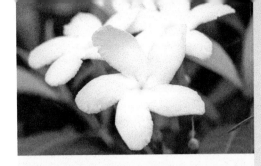

PRECAUTIONS

Because it can stimulate menstrual flow, pregnant women should avoid jasmine essential oil.

- Do not use if you are pregnant.

IMPROVE CONCENTRATION WHILE FRESHENING INDOOR AIR NATURALLY. A Japanese study found that mental concentration and accuracy improved when jasmine essential oil was diffused in an office environment, decreasing errors by 33 percent. Lemon essential oil proved even more effective, decreasing mistakes by 54 percent. Lavender essential oil helped, too, decreasing errors by 20 percent.

MEDICINAL USES

Acne

Addiction

Antibacterial

Aphrodisiac

Breastfeeding

Childbirth

Depression

Expectorant

Fatigue

Hepatitis

Impotence

Low testosterone

Menstrual support

Muscle pain and stiffness

Nervousness

PMS

Relaxation

Respiratory ailments

Scarring

Skin care

Stress

Stretch marks

Juniper *Juniperus communis*

Drive through nearly any neighborhood or visit a public park, and you are likely to encounter a juniper tree or two. These fragrant conifers have been used for spiritual and medicinal purposes since ancient times, and they continue to prove useful today. Juniper essential oil is excellent for treating muscle pain and a variety of skin conditions, and its deeply calming fragrance helps evaporate stress.

APPLICATION METHODS

- Use in the bath or shower for absorption and aromatherapy benefits
- Diffuse for aromatherapy benefits
- Massage, diluted, for physical ailments
- Use with compress for muscle pain and stiffness

BLENDS WITH

- Bay
- Benzoin
- Bergamot
- Black pepper
- Carrot seed
- Cedarwood
- Clary sage
- Cypress
- Elemi
- Eucalyptus
- Fennel
- Geranium
- Ginger
- Grapefruit
- Helichrysum
- Lavender
- Lemon
- Lemon eucalyptus
- Mandarin
- Marjoram
- Myrrh
- Neroli
- Orange
- Palmarosa
- Peppermint
- Petitgrain
- Pine
- Rose geranium
- Rosemary
- Spikenard
- Tangerine
- Tea tree

PRECAUTIONS

Those with kidney or liver disease should avoid juniper essential oil. Because it can stimulate menstrual flow, pregnant women should avoid juniper essential oil.

- Do not use if you are pregnant.
- Do not use if you have kidney disease.
- Do not use if you have liver disease.
- Not safe for children under 6.

SPEED WOUND HEALING WITH JUNIPER.
An exciting study reported in the January 2013 issue of *Journal of Medicinal Food* focused on the ability of juniper essential oil to speed wound healing. Both *juniperus virginiana* and *juniperus occidentalis* were shown to reduce inflammation and help wounds heal faster.

MEDICINAL USES

Acne	Insect repellant
Addiction	Meditation
Analgesic	Menstrual
Anti-	support
inflammatory	Muscle pain
Antimicrobial	and stiffness
Antiseptic	Nervousness
Anxiety	Prostatitis
Arthritis	Psoriasis
Calming	Rheumatism
Cellulite	Sedative
Diuretic	Skin care
Eczema	Stress
Fatigue	Weight-loss
Gout	support
Hangover	Wounds

Lavandin *Lavandula hybrida*

Lavandin is sometimes confused for lavender, and for good reason: It is a hybrid plant that was developed by crossing lavender with aspic. Grown largely for the perfume industry, it is not as medicinally valuable as lavender; however, lavandin essential oil is useful for a number of applications, including dermatitis, joint and muscle pain and stiffness, and stress.

APPLICATION METHODS

- Use in the bath or shower for absorption and aromatherapy benefits
- Diffuse for aromatherapy benefits
- Massage, diluted, for physical ailments
- Use with compress for muscle pain and stiffness

BLENDS WITH

- Bergamot
- Cinnamon
- Citronella
- Clary sage
- Jasmine
- Patchouli
- Pine
- Rosemary
- Sage
- Thyme

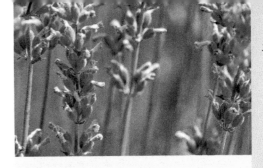

PRECAUTIONS

Lavandin essential oil is generally considered safe.

RELIEVE ANXIETY BEFORE SURGERY WITH LAVANDIN ESSENTIAL OIL. Lavandin essential oil has been proven to positively affect patients who are experiencing preoperative anxiety, eliminating the need for medications that could negatively impact recovery. A study published in the 2009 *Journal of PeriAnesthesia Nursing* shows significantly lower levels of anxiety in patients in a lavandin essential oil group than those patients who received standard medications.

MEDICINAL USES

Analgesic

Antidepressant

Antiseptic

Blister

Boil

Circulatory health

Cold

Cough

Dermatitis

Expectorant

Flu

Insect bites

Joint pain

Lice

Muscle pain and stiffness

Relaxation

Scabies

Stress

Vertigo

Wounds

Lavender *Lavandula angustifolia*

If you must choose just one essential oil to begin with, lavender may be the best choice. Probably the most versatile of all essential oils, it blends well with many others, treats an astonishingly wide array of physical ailments, and can make a positive difference emotionally. It may also be used in formulating nontoxic household cleaners, laundry detergent, deodorant, and much more.

APPLICATION METHODS

- Use in the bath or shower for absorption and aromatherapy benefits
- Diffuse for aromatherapy benefits
- Massage, diluted, for physical ailments
- Use with compress for muscle pain and stiffness

BLENDS WITH

- Basil
- Bay
- Benzoin
- Bergamot
- Black pepper
- Cajeput
- Calamus
- Camphor
- Caraway
- Carrot seed
- Cedarwood
- Cinnamon
- Citronella
- Clary sage
- Clove
- Cypress
- Elemi
- Eucalyptus
- Fennel
- Fir needle
- Frankincense
- Geranium
- German chamomile
- Grapefruit
- Helichrysum
- Hyssop
- Juniper
- Lemon
- Lemon eucalyptus
- Lemongrass
- Lime
- Mandarin
- Manuka
- Marjoram
- Melissa
- Myrrh
- Neroli
- Niaouli
- Nutmeg

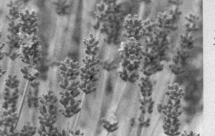

- Orange
- Oregano
- Palmarosa
- Patchouli
- Peppermint
- Petitgrain
- Pine
- Roman chamomile
- Rose
- Rose geranium
- Rosemary
- Sage
- Sandalwood
- Spearmint
- Spikenard
- Spruce
- Tagetes
- Tea tree
- Thyme
- Valerian
- Vetiver

PRECAUTIONS

Those with an estrogen-dependent cancer should avoid lavender essential oil. Lavender essential oil has a deeply relaxing effect and should not be used prior to driving, operating machinery, or doing other tasks that require concentration.

- Do not use if you have an estrogen-dependent cancer.
- May act as a sedative.

MEDICINAL USES

Acne	Hypertension
Analgesic	Insect bites
Antiallergenic	Insecticide
Antibacterial	Insect repellent
Anti-inflammatory	Insomnia
	Irritability
Antimicrobial	Itchiness
Antiseptic	Lice
Anxiety	Migraine
Asthma	Muscle pain
Athlete's foot	and stiffness
Boil	Nausea
Bruise	Nightmares
Burn	Rheumatism
Chicken pox	Scabies
Chilblains	Sedative
Childbirth	Sprains and
Colic	strains
Dandruff	Stress
Depression	Stretch marks
Dermatitis	Sunburn
Diuretic	Vomiting
Earache	Whooping
Flatulence	cough
Headache	Wounds

Lemon   *Citrus limon*

Lemon is a powerful detoxification agent, it contains high levels of vitamins and minerals, and its flavor and scent are appreciated worldwide. Lemon essential oil takes the power of lemon to new heights, and it can be used to treat illnesses, improve mood, and boost alertness.

APPLICATION METHODS

- Use in the bath or shower for absorption and aromatherapy benefits
- Diffuse for aromatherapy benefits
- Massage, diluted, for physical ailments
- Use with compress for muscle pain and stiffness

BLENDS WITH

- Basil
- Bay
- Benzoin
- Birch
- Black pepper
- Camphor
- Cardamom
- Carrot seed
- Cedarwood
- Cinnamon
- Citronella
- Clove
- Coriander
- Dill
- Eucalyptus
- Fennel
- Fir needle
- Frankincense
- Geranium
- German chamomile
- Ginger
- Grapefruit
- Helichrysum
- Hyssop
- Jasmine
- Juniper
- Lavender
- Lemongrass
- Lemon verbena
- Mandarin
- Manuka
- Marjoram
- Melissa
- Myrrh
- Neroli
- Niaouli
- Orange
- Oregano
- Palmarosa
- Peppermint
- Petitgrain
- Roman chamomile

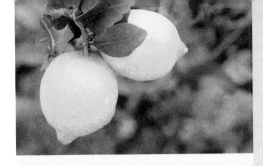

- Rose
- Rose geranium
- Rosemary
- Rosewood
- Sage
- Sandalwood
- Spearmint
- Spikenard
- Tagetes
- Tangerine
- Tea tree
- Thyme
- Vetiver
- Ylang-ylang

PRECAUTIONS

Lemon essential oil can be a dermal irritant for sensitive individuals. Conduct a patch test before use. It is also phototoxic. Avoid exposing application sites to sunlight for 12 to 24 hours following application. Lemon essential oil has a short shelf life in comparison with other essential oils; use it within eight to ten months of purchase to ensure freshness.

- Avoid exposure to sunlight for 12 to 24 hours after use.
- May cause skin irritation.
- Use within 8 to 10 months of purchase date.

COMBAT CANDIDA WITH LEMON ESSENTIAL OIL.

In a 2014 study published in the journal *Mycopathologia*, lemon essential oil was proven effective against candida, which are opportunistic fungi that can cause severe infections in people with compromised immune systems. Eucalyptus, cinnamon, and pine essential oils were also shown effective in combating these fungi.

MEDICINAL USES

Acne	Fever
Antibacterial	Flu
Antifungal	Headache
Anti-inflammatory	Hypertension
	Indigestion
Antimicrobial	Insecticide
Antiseptic	Insect repellent
Arthritis	Laxative
Boil	Mental alertness
Bronchitis	
Canker sore	Migraine
Cellulite	Nosebleed
Chilblains	Sore throat
Cold	Varicose veins
Constipation	Wart
Corns	Wounds
Diuretic	

Lemon Eucalyptus   *Eucalyptus citriodora*

Like its close relative eucalyptus, lemon eucalyptus proves useful for a wide range of applications, ranging from eliminating cigarette smoke odor to helping alleviate symptoms associated with respiratory illness. It is useful as an insect repellent, eases arthritis pain, improves circulation, and much more.

APPLICATION METHODS

- Use in the bath or shower for absorption and aromatherapy benefits
- Diffuse for aromatherapy benefits
- Massage, diluted, for physical ailments
- Use with compress for muscle pain and stiffness

BLENDS WITH

- Basil
- Black pepper
- Cedarwood
- Clary sage
- Clove
- Cypress
- Eucalyptus
- Frankincense
- Geranium
- Ginger
- Juniper
- Lavender
- Marjoram
- Orange
- Peppermint
- Pine
- Rose geranium
- Rosemary
- Sage
- Tea tree
- Thyme
- Vetiver
- Ylang-ylang

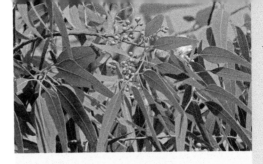

PRECAUTIONS

Lemon eucalyptus essential oil is generally considered safe.

ENJOY THE OUTSIDE BUG-FREE WITH LEMON EUCALYPTUS. Lemon eucalyptus essential oil is one of the most effective mosquito, gnat, and biting fly repellents available. Many people are concerned about the health effects of the heavy use of DEET but since it is considered to be an effective product, there seemed like no compelling alternative. In trials in Tanzania, lemon eucalyptus essential oil was found to confer complete mosquito repellent protection for six to eight hours.

MEDICINAL USES

Acne

Antibacterial

Antifungal

Antiseptic

Antiviral

Arthritis

Calming

Chicken pox

Cold

Cough

Circulatory health

Emphysema

Expectorant

Flu

Insecticide

Insect repellent

Measles

Rheumatism

Sinus infection

Lemongrass *Cymbopogon flexuosus, C. citratus*

Lemongrass is a popular ingredient in savory foods, and its medicinal use is sometimes overlooked completely. Sourced from a humble tropical grass, lemongrass essential oil has a fresh, enticing fragrance that revitalizes mind and body. It is useful for a surprising number of applications, ranging from repelling ticks, fleas, and other insects to helping injured ligaments heal faster.

APPLICATION METHODS

- Use in the bath or shower for absorption and aromatherapy benefits
- Diffuse for aromatherapy benefits
- Massage, diluted, for physical ailments
- Use with compress for muscle pain and stiffness

BLENDS WITH

- Basil
- Bergamot
- Black pepper
- Cardamom
- Cedarwood
- Clary sage
- Coriander
- Cypress
- Fennel
- Geranium
- Ginger
- Grapefruit
- Lavender
- Lemon
- Marjoram
- Orange
- Palmarosa
- Patchouli
- Rosemary
- Tea tree
- Thyme
- Vetiver
- Ylang-ylang

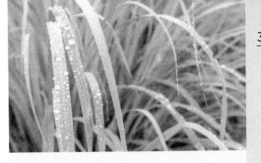

PRECAUTIONS

Lemongrass essential oil can be a dermal irritant for sensitive individuals. Conduct a patch test before use. Those with an estrogen-dependent cancer should avoid lemongrass essential oil.

- Do not use if you have an estrogen-dependent cancer.
- May cause skin irritation.
- Not safe for children under 6.

FIGHT INFECTION WITH LEMONGRASS. According to a study published in the November 2012 issue of the *Journal of Applied Microbiology*, lemongrass essential oil exhibits a high level of antimicrobial activity. This natural remedy is so powerful that it is able to combat antibiotic-resistant Staphylococcus aureus (staph).

MEDICINAL USES

Analgesic	Fleas
Antifungal	Flu
Anti-inflammatory	Fungicidal
Antimicrobial	Headache
Antiseptic	Insecticide
Antiviral	Insect repellent
Athlete's foot	Jet lag
Bactericidal	Jock itch
Cellulite	Lice
Circulatory health	Muscle pain and stiffness
Cold	Scabies
Cough	Tendinitis
Detoxification	Tennis elbow
Flatulence	Ticks
	Varicose veins

Lemon Verbena   *Lippia citrodora, Aloysia triphylla*

Lemon verbena is a deciduous shrub native to Chile and Argentina and now culti-vated in many parts of the world. The plant gets its name from its sweet, lemon-fresh aroma, and essential oil sourced from its freshly harvested leaves has the ability to boost mood, soften skin, and aid in hangover recovery.

APPLICATION METHODS

- Use in the bath or shower for absorption and aromatherapy benefits
- Diffuse for aromatherapy benefits
- Massage, diluted, for physical ailments

BLENDS WITH

- Basil
- Elemi
- Lemon
- Neroli
- Palmarosa

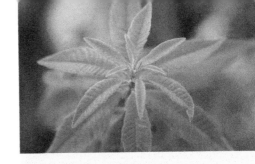

PRECAUTIONS

Lemon verbena essential oil is phototoxic.

- Avoid exposure to sunlight for 12 to 24 hours after use.

TREAT DIGESTIVE AILMENTS NATURALLY WITH LEMON VERBENA. Many digestive ailments are complicated by bacterial overgrowth. One pathogen that contributes to gastric disease is H. pylori, a microbe that is becoming increasingly resistant to antibiotics. In a clinical study, lemon verbena essential oil was shown effective against the bacteria even after it had developed resistance to the antibiotic clarithromycin.

MEDICINAL USES

Alcoholism

Antiseptic

Aphrodisiac

Bronchitis

Cramping

Cirrhosis

Decongestant

Depression

Emotional balance

Fever

Fluid retention

Hangover

Healthy liver function

Indigestion

Insecticide

Insect repellant

Nervousness

Relaxation

Sedative

Skin care

Stress

Lime *Citrus aurantiifolia*

With its vibrant green skin and its fresh, tangy taste, lime is a favorite with people everywhere. Lime essential oil captures lime's best qualities; its scent is irresistible, and its ability to eliminate moodiness is nearly legendary. Use lime essential oil as a natural air freshener or to treat arthritis, fever, insect bites, and other ailments.

APPLICATION METHODS

- Use in the bath or shower for absorption and aromatherapy benefits
- Diffuse for aromatherapy benefits
- Massage, diluted, for physical ailments
- Use with compress for muscle pain and stiffness

BLENDS WITH

- Black pepper
- Carrot seed
- Citronella
- Clary sage
- Dill
- Ginger
- Jasmine
- Lavender
- Neroli
- Nutmeg
- Rose geranium
- Rosemary
- Rosewood
- Ylang-ylang

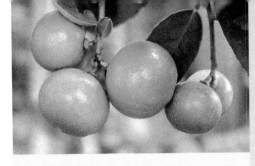

PRECAUTIONS

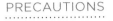

Lime essential oil can be a dermal irritant for sensitive individuals. Conduct a patch test before use. It is phototoxic. Avoid exposing application sites to sunlight for 12 to 24 hours following application.

- Avoid exposure to sunlight for 12 to 24 hours after use.
- May cause skin irritation.

MEDICINAL USES

Acne	Fever
Antibacterial	Indoor air
Antiseptic	freshener
Antiviral	Insect bites
Arthritis	Joint pain
Bactericidal	Mental
Bronchitis	alertness
Cellulite	Muscle pain
Chilblains	and stiffness
Circulatory	Oily hair
health	Oily skin
Cold	Rheumatism
Cold sore	Sinus infection
Cough	Stress
Depression	Varicose veins
Fatigue	Wounds

Mandarin *Citrus reticulata*

If you have young children, mandarin essential oil is one of the best essential oils to keep on hand for calming tired minds, soothing temper tantrums, and easing insomnia. Its bright, cheery fragrance makes it ideal for use as a natural air freshener, and its ability to alleviate a number of common skin problems makes it a great choice for use in skin care preparations.

APPLICATION METHODS

- Use in the bath or shower for absorption and aromatherapy benefits
- Diffuse for aromatherapy benefits
- Massage, diluted, for physical ailments
- Use with compress for muscle pain and stiffness

BLENDS WITH

- Aniseed
- Basil
- Bergamot
- Black pepper
- Cardamom
- Cinnamon
- Clary sage
- Clove
- Fennel
- Frankincense
- Geranium
- Ginger
- Grapefruit
- Hyssop
- Jasmine
- Juniper
- Lavender
- Lemon
- Myrrh
- Neroli
- Nutmeg
- Palmarosa
- Patchouli
- Petitgrain
- Roman chamomile
- Rose
- Rose geranium
- Sandalwood
- Valerian
- Vetiver
- Ylang-ylang

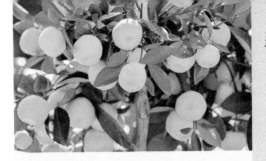

PRECAUTIONS

Mandarin essential oil is phototoxic.

- Avoid exposure to sunlight for 12 to 24 hours after use.

MEDICINAL USES

Acne	Mood booster
Antimicrobial	Nervousness
Antiseptic	Oily hair
Cold	Oily skin
Constipation	Scars
Cough	Sedative
Diarrhea	Skin care
Disinfectant	Stimulant
Diuretic	Stress
Flatulence	Stretch marks
Flu	Temper
Hypnotic	tantrums
Insomnia	Tension
Laxative	Wrinkles

Manuka   *Leptospermum scoparium*

New Zealand natives have used Manuka for millennia, incorporating it into treatments for a wide range of illnesses and enjoying it in relaxing tea. Manuka essential oil is relatively new to aromatherapy, but don't let that stop you from using it to treat common ailments like dandruff, insect bites, swimmer's ear, and more.

APPLICATION METHODS

- Use in the bath or shower for absorption and aromatherapy benefits
- Diffuse for aromatherapy benefits
- Massage, diluted, for physical ailments
- Use with compress for muscle pain and stiffness

BLENDS WITH

- Basil
- Bergamot
- Black pepper
- Clary sage
- Cypress
- Eucalyptus
- Geranium
- German chamomile
- Grapefruit
- Lavender
- Lemon
- Marjoram
- Orange
- Patchouli
- Peppermint
- Petitgrain
- Pine
- Roman chamomile
- Rosemary
- Sage
- Sandalwood
- Tea tree
- Thyme

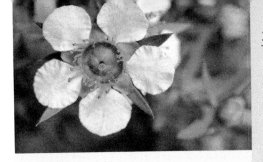

PRECAUTIONS

- Not safe for internal use.

PROTECT YOURSELF FROM BACTERIA WITH MANUKA ESSENTIAL OIL. Antibiotic-resistant bacteria are a serious concern because treatment can be ineffective and the results deadly. Laboratory tests have shown that Manuka essential oil is effective so far against 39 microorganisms including the bacteria that causes acne, staphylococcal bacteria, streptococci, and even MRSA (Methicillin-Resistant Staph. Aureus) bacteria, which shows no effects from antibiotics. Manuka essential oil has anti-fungal and anti-inflammatory properties as well, making it a good treatment for skin infections.

MEDICINAL USES

Analgesic	Expectorant
Anesthetic	Flu
Anger	Immune
Antiallergenic	stimulant
Antibacterial	Insect bites
Antifungal	Insect repellant
Anti-	Jock itch
inflammatory	Nervousness
Antimicrobial	Scarring
Antiseptic	Sedative
Antiviral	Sinus infection
Anxiety	Spider bites
Athlete's foot	Stretch marks
Cold	Swimmer's ear
Cough	Tick bites
Dandruff	Wounds

Marjoram   *Origanum majorana, Marjorana hortensis*

Marjoram is a very popular culinary ingredient with an interesting history; ancient Greeks gave it to newlywed couples to assure good fortune. Essential oil made with this humble herb has a lovely, warm smell with spicy undertones. It is particularly useful in treating pain, easing respiratory complaints, and bringing emotional balance.

APPLICATION METHODS

- Use in the bath or shower for absorption and aromatherapy benefits
- Diffuse for aromatherapy benefits
- Massage, diluted, for physical ailments
- Use with compress for muscle pain and stiffness

BLENDS WITH

- Basil
- Bergamot
- Black pepper
- Cedarwood
- Cinnamon
- Cypress
- Eucalyptus
- Fennel
- Fir needle
- German chamomile
- Juniper
- Lavender
- Lemon
- Lemon eucalyptus
- Lemongrass
- Manuka
- Orange
- Peppermint
- Petitgrain
- Pine
- Rosemary
- Tea tree
- Thyme

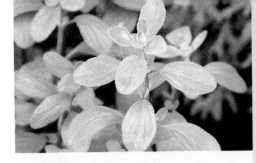

PRECAUTIONS

Because it can stimulate menstrual flow, pregnant women should avoid marjoram essential oil. Marjoram essential oil has a deeply relaxing effect and should not be used prior to driving, operating machinery, or doing other tasks that require concentration.

- Do not use if you are pregnant.
- May act as a sedative.

MEDICINAL USES

ADD/ADHD	Grief
Analgesic	Headache
Antiseptic	Indigestion
Antiviral	Joint pain
Anxiety	Laxative
Arthritis	Menstrual
Asthma	support
Bronchitis	Migraine
Bruise	Muscle pain
Chilblains	and stiffness
Circulatory	Relaxation
health	Rheumatism
Cold	Sedative
Cough	Sinus infection
Diuretic	Sprains and
Expectorant	strains
Flu	Stress

Melissa   *Melissa officinalis*

Also known as sweet balm and lemon balm, melissa has been used to treat a number of physical and emotional ailments since ancient times. Like the herb from which it is derived, melissa essential oil brings calm to troubled minds and has a positive effect on a wide range of ailments, including fungal infections, cold sores, and hypertension.

APPLICATION METHODS

- Use in the bath or shower for absorption and aromatherapy benefits
- Diffuse for aromatherapy benefits
- Massage, diluted, for physical ailments
- Use with a compress for muscle pain and stiffness

BLENDS WITH

- Bergamot
- Camphor
- Frankincense
- Geranium
- German chamomile
- Lavender
- Lemon
- Neroli
- Orange
- Petitgrain
- Roman chamomile
- Rose

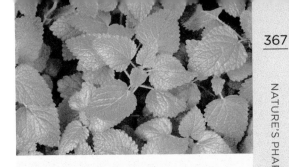

PRECAUTIONS

Melissa essential oil can be a dermal irritant for sensitive individuals. Conduct a patch test before use. Use a low dilution rate. Because it can stimulate menstrual flow, pregnant women should avoid melissa essential oil.

- Do not use if you are pregnant.
- May cause skin irritation.

FIGHT COLD SORES WITH MELISSA ESSENTIAL OIL.
Melissa essential oil has been proven to be a potent antiviral agent, and a 2012 study reported by the journal *Chemotherapy* showed that this essential oil inhibits the growth of herpes simplex even when applied at low concentrations.

MEDICINAL USES

Antiallergenic

Antibacterial

Antifungal

Anti-inflammatory

Antiseptic

Antiviral

Bactericidal

Calming

Cold sore

Depression

Fever

Flatulence

Hair growth

Headache

Herpes

Hypertension

Indigestion

Menstrual support

Nausea

Nervousness

Sedative

Stress

Myrrh *Commiphora myrrha*

Myrrh was a luxury item in the ancient world, used in embalming Egyptian royalty and given as a gift of esteem to the infant Jesus. Today anyone can enjoy the fragrance and health benefits myrrh offers; this delightful essential oil is effective in addressing emotional and physical complaints, treating problem skin, and even improving dental health.

APPLICATION METHODS

- Use in the bath or shower for absorption and aromatherapy benefits
- Diffuse for aromatherapy benefits
- Gargle for dental health and halitosis
- Massage, diluted, for physical ailments
- Use with compress for muscle pain and stiffness

BLENDS WITH

- Benzoin
- Bergamot
- Clove
- Cypress
- Elemi
- Frankincense
- Geranium
- German chamomile
- Grapefruit
- Jasmine
- Juniper
- Lavender
- Lemon
- Neroli
- Orange
- Palmarosa
- Patchouli
- Pine
- Roman chamomile
- Rose
- Rose geranium
- Rosemary
- Sandalwood
- Spikenard
- Tangerine
- Tea tree
- Vetiver
- Ylang-ylang

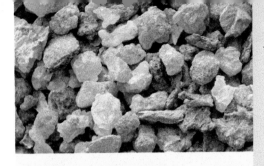

PRECAUTIONS

Do not use myrrh essential oil internally. Because it can stimulate menstrual flow, pregnant women should avoid myrrh essential oil.

- Do not use if you are pregnant.
- Not safe for internal use.

MEDICINAL USES

Antifungal

Anti-inflammatory

Antimicrobial

Antiseptic

Antiviral

Athlete's foot

Bronchitis

Dental health

Diarrhea

Dysentery

Expectorant

Fungicidal

Halitosis

Hemorrhoids

Hyperthyroidism

Meditation

Ringworm

Sedative

Skin care

Stretch marks

Ulcers

Wounds

Wrinkles

Neroli   *Citrus aurantium*

A single pound of neroli essential oil contains about 1,000 pounds of freshly harvested orange blossoms, which explains why this intoxicating essential oil is one of the more costly to obtain. Because of its ability to alleviate depression, ease anxiety, address menstrual and premenstrual issues, and soften skin, it is well worth the investment.

APPLICATION METHODS

- Use in the bath or shower for absorption and aromatherapy benefits
- Diffuse for aromatherapy benefits
- Massage, diluted, for physical ailments
- Use with compress for muscle pain and stiffness

BLENDS WITH

- Allspice
- Basil
- Benzoin
- Bergamot
- Cardamom
- Cedarwood
- Clary sage
- Coriander
- Frankincense
- Geranium
- German chamomile
- Ginger
- Grapefruit
- Helichrysum
- Jasmine
- Juniper
- Lavender
- Lemon
- Lemon verbena
- Lime
- Mandarin
- Melissa
- Myrrh
- Orange
- Palmarosa
- Patchouli
- Petitgrain
- Roman chamomile
- Rose geranium
- Sandalwood
- Spikenard
- Tangerine
- Ylang-ylang

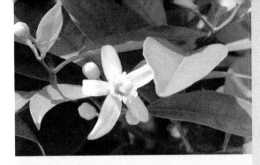

PRECAUTIONS

Neroli essential oil has a deeply relaxing effect and should not be used prior to driving, operating machinery, or doing other tasks that require concentration.

- May act as a sedative.

STOP STRESS WITH A NEROLI ESSENTIAL OIL BLEND. According to a study published in the journal *Evidence-Based Complementary and Alternative Medicine*, a group of hypertensive and pre-hypertensive test subjects were treated to an aromatherapy blend containing 20 percent lavender essential oil, 15 percent ylang-ylang essential oil, 10 percent marjoram essential oil, and 2 percent neroli essential oil. While their nighttime blood pressure numbers didn't decrease, their daytime blood pressure numbers dropped, as did their reported stress levels.

MEDICINAL USES

Aging skin	Heart
Antibacterial	palpitations
Anti-	Hypertension
inflammatory	Insomnia
Antiseptic	Menstrual
Antiviral	support
Anxiety	PMS
Aphrodisiac	Pregnancy
Broken or	Rosacea
swollen	Scarring
capillaries	Sedative
Circulatory	Shock
health	Stress
Depression	Stretch marks
Fungicidal	Vertigo
Headache	Wrinkles

Niaouli   *Melaleuca viridiflora, M. quinquenervia*

Like its close relative tea tree, niaouli offers a wide range of benefits. This essential oil has a fresh, slightly sweet fragrance that most people enjoy, and its antiseptic power makes it a popular ingredient in oral health preparations such as toothpaste and breath spray.

APPLICATION METHODS

- Use in the bath or shower for absorption and aromatherapy benefits
- Diffuse for aromatherapy benefits
- Massage, diluted, for physical ailments
- Use with compress for muscle pain and stiffness

BLENDS WITH

- Bergamot
- Eucalyptus
- Fennel
- Lavender
- Lemon
- Orange
- Peppermint
- Rosemary
- Tea tree

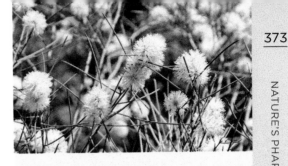

PRECAUTIONS

Niaouli essential oil is generally considered safe.

BOOST YOUR IMMUNE SYSTEM WITH NIAOULI ESSENTIAL OIL. Samples of niaouli essential oil were brought back to England from Australia in 1770 by Captain Cook after naturalists observed Aborigines using it for cuts, infections, pain, and other health concerns. Niaouli essential oil can be used undiluted to help fight bacterial infections and boost the immune system. This essential oil can increase white blood cells and antibodies. Some hospitals use Niaouli during cobalt radiation therapy for cancer to lessen the severity of associated burns and promote quicker healing.

MEDICINAL USES

Acne

Analgesic

Anti-inflammatory

Antiseptic

Bactericidal

Boil

Burn

Cold

Cough

Expectorant

Fever

Flu

Insect bites

Insect repellent

Intestinal parasites

Mental alertness

Oily hair

Oily skin

Rheumatism

Sinus infection

Sore throat

Urinary tract infection

Whooping cough

Wounds

Nutmeg   *Myristica fragrans*

Nutmeg is a favorite in kitchens everywhere, but its essential oil benefits extend to treating a wide range of ailments, ranging from indigestion to muscle pain and stiffness. Its spicy aroma is pleasing to most, and its ability to stimulate the mind while freshening air naturally makes it a good choice for diffusing, particularly in blends with other essential oils.

APPLICATION METHODS

- Use in the bath or shower for absorption and aromatherapy benefits
- Diffuse for aromatherapy benefits
- Massage, diluted, for physical ailments
- Use with compress for muscle pain and stiffness

BLENDS WITH

- Bay
- Bergamot
- Black pepper
- Camphor
- Carrot seed
- Cassia
- Cinnamon
- Clary sage
- Coriander
- Dill
- Geranium
- Lavender
- Lime
- Mandarin
- Orange
- Petitgrain
- Rosemary
- Tangerine
- Tea tree

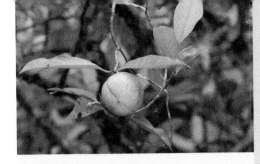

PRECAUTIONS

Do not use nutmeg essential oil internally. Because it can stimulate menstrual flow, pregnant women should avoid nutmeg essential oil. Those with cancer should avoid using it as well. Nutmeg essential oil has a deeply relaxing effect and should not be used prior to driving, operating machinery, or doing other tasks that require concentration.

- Do not use if you are pregnant.
- Do not use if you have cancer.
- May act as a sedative.
- Not safe for internal use.

MEDICINAL USES

Analgesic

Antiseptic

Aphrodisiac

Arthritis

Circulatory health

Gallstones

Gout

Heart health

Indigestion

Laxative

Mental alertness

Muscle pain and stiffness

Rheumatism

Orange *Citrus sinensis*

Many increase their consumption of oranges during cold and flu season. Take advantage of orange essential oil's ability to help mitigate common symptoms of these ailments, and you are likely to find that you feel better overall. This simple, fragrant essential oil also imparts feelings of warmth and happiness while helping to eliminate toxins and address a wide range of common ailments.

APPLICATION METHODS

- Use in the bath or shower for absorption and aromatherapy benefits
- Diffuse for aromatherapy benefits
- Massage, diluted, for physical ailments
- Use with compress for muscle pain and stiffness

BLENDS WITH

- Allspice
- Basil
- Bay
- Benzoin
- Bergamot
- Birch
- Black pepper
- Camphor
- Caraway
- Cardamom
- Carrot seed
- Cinnamon
- Citronella
- Clary sage
- Clove
- Coriander
- Dill
- Eucalyptus
- Fennel
- Fir needle
- Frankincense
- Geranium
- Ginger
- Grapefruit
- Helichrysum
- Hyssop
- Jasmine
- Juniper
- Lavender
- Lemon
- Lemon eucalyptus
- Lemongrass
- Manuka
- Marjoram
- Melissa
- Myrrh
- Neroli
- Niaouli
- Nutmeg

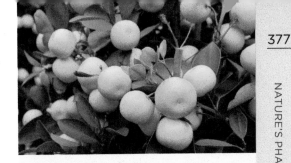

- Oregano
- Palmarosa
- Patchouli
- Petitgrain
- Rose
- Rose geranium
- Rosewood
- Sandalwood
- Spearmint
- Tagetes
- Vetiver
- Ylang-ylang

PRECAUTIONS

Orange essential oil is phototoxic. Avoid exposing application sites to sunlight for 12 to 24 hours following application. Orange essential oil has a very short shelf life, generally just about six months.

- Avoid exposure to sunlight for 12 to 24 hours after use.
- Use within 6 months of purchase date.

REDUCE FEAR AND ANXIETY NATURALLY WITH ORANGE ESSENTIAL OIL. Orange essential oil is an excellent addition to your regimen, particularly if you suffer from fear or anxiety. In a 2013 study published by *Advanced Biomedical Research*, children who inhaled orange essential oil while undergoing dental procedures showed fewer physical manifestations associated with fear and anxiety.

MEDICINAL USES

Acne

Aging skin

Anti-inflammatory

Antiseptic

Bactericidal

Cold

Constipation

Dermatitis

Diuretic

Expectorant

Flu

Fungicidal

Immune stimulant

Insomnia

Irritability

Nervousness

Stress

Oregano   *Origanum vulgare*

Oregano gives many Mediterranean dishes their delectable flavors and aromas. This humble herb has potent healing effects, too, particularly when used to formulate essential oil. Its antibacterial, antiviral, and immune-stimulating properties make it useful in combating infections.

APPLICATION METHODS

- Diffuse for aromatherapy benefits
- Massage, diluted, for muscle pain and stiffness

BLENDS WITH

- Bay
- Bergamot
- Camphor
- Cedarwood
- Citronella
- Cypress
- Eucalyptus
- German chamomile
- Lavender
- Lemon
- Orange
- Petitgrain
- Pine
- Roman chamomile
- Rosemary
- Tea tree
- Thyme

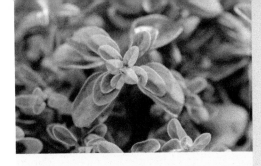

PRECAUTIONS

Oregano essential oil can be a dermal irritant for sensitive individuals. Conduct a patch test before use. Oregano essential oil irritates the mucus membranes. Because it can stimulate menstrual flow, pregnant women should avoid oregano essential oil.

- Avoid contact with mucus membranes.
- Do not use if you are pregnant.
- May cause skin irritation.

MEDICINAL USES

Abscess

Analgesic

Antibacterial

Antifungal

Antimicrobial

Antiseptic

Antiviral

Arthritis

Boil

Bronchitis

Cold

Cough

Diuretic

Expectorant

Flu

Immune stimulant

Pneumonia

Radiation damage

Rheumatism

Strep throat

Ticks

Typhoid fever

Whooping cough

Yeast infection

Palmarosa   *Cymbopogon martinii*

If you suffer from dry skin, be sure to add palmarosa essential oil to your arsenal of natural remedies. This sweet, rose-scented essential oil is extracted from a wild grass with flowering tops, and is a popular ingredient in cosmetics, soaps, and perfumes. In addition to its value as a skin softener, it has a number of medicinal uses.

APPLICATION METHODS

- Use in the bath or shower for absorption and aromatherapy benefits
- Diffuse for aromatherapy benefits
- Massage, diluted, for physical ailments
- Neat for athlete's foot
- Use with compress for muscle pain and stiffness

BLENDS WITH

- Bay
- Bergamot
- Cardamom
- Cedarwood
- Clary sage
- Clove
- Coriander
- Frankincense
- Geranium
- German chamomile
- Ginger
- Grapefruit
- Helichrysum
- Juniper
- Lavender
- Lemon
- Lemongrass
- Mandarin
- Myrrh
- Neroli
- Orange
- Patchouli
- Petitgrain
- Roman chamomile
- Rose
- Rose geranium
- Sandalwood
- Spikenard
- Tangerine
- Ylang-ylang

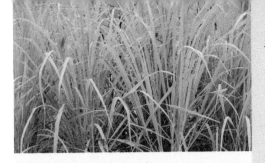

PRECAUTIONS

Palmarosa essential oil is generally considered safe.

BANISH BACTERIA WITH PALMAROSA.
In a 2009 study reported by the Indian *Journal of Pharmaceutical Sciences*, palmarosa essential oil was proven to exhibit activity against both gram-positive and gram-negative bacteria. While lavender and tuberose essential oils were also studied, palmarosa essential oil showed the highest activity against the bacteria among the three essential oils.

MEDICINAL USES

Acne
Antibacterial
Antifungal
Antiseptic
Antiviral
Athlete's foot
Calming
Dermatitis
Fatigue
Fever
Indigestion
Mental alertness
Muscle pain and stiffness
Scarring
Skin care
Stress

Patchouli *Pogostemon cablin*

The warm, rich fragrance of patchouli reminds many people of the 1960s and '70s, but its usefulness extends far beyond the creation of seductive perfumes and incense blends. Valuable for treating a wide range of skin conditions, easing fever, and creating natural insect repellent, it is an excellent addition to your collection of essential oils. Don't worry about whether you'll be able to use it up before its shelf life is over; unlike most essential oils, patchouli improves with age.

APPLICATION METHODS

- Use in the bath or shower for absorption and aromatherapy benefits
- Diffuse for aromatherapy benefits
- Massage, diluted, for physical ailments
- Neat for athlete's foot and insect bites
- Use with compress for muscle pain and stiffness

BLENDS WITH

- Allspice
- Bay
- Bergamot
- Black pepper
- Calamus
- Cardamom
- Cedarwood
- Cinnamon
- Clary sage
- Clove
- Coriander
- Frankincense
- Geranium
- German chamomile
- Ginger
- Grapefruit
- Jasmine
- Lavandin
- Lavender
- Lemongrass
- Mandarin
- Manuka
- Myrrh
- Neroli
- Orange
- Palmarosa
- Petitgrain
- Roman chamomile
- Rose
- Rose geranium
- Sandalwood
- Spikenard
- Tangerine
- Valerian
- Vetiver
- Ylang-ylang

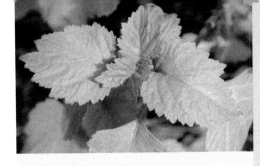

PRECAUTIONS

Patchouli essential oil is generally considered safe.

SLEEP SOUNDLY AND KEEP THE BED BUGS AWAY WITH PATCHOULI OIL. Patchouli essential oil infused imported cashmere shawls with its scent en route to England in Victorian times, and ladies of fashion would not buy the shawls without this signature fragrance. The oil was placed between the shawls to prevent moths from damaging the expensive merchandise, not as a scent. In 2005, a study in *Phytotherapy Research* proved that patchouli oil also repels other bugs such as mosquitos and bed bugs. Placing the satchels in beds to keep bed bugs away also helps promote sleep. This sedative effect was outlined in a 2011 study in the *Journal of Natural Medicines*.

MEDICINAL USES

Acne

Antibacterial

Anti-inflammatory

Antimicrobial

Antiseptic

Antiviral

Anxiety

Aphrodisiac

Appetite suppressant

Athlete's foot

Bactericidal

Cellulite

Decongestant

Depression

Dermatitis

Diuretic

Eczema

Emotional balance

Fever

Insect bites

Insect repellant

Laxative

Meditation

Scarring

Skin care

Peppermint *Mentha x piperita*

With its clean, crisp fragrance and its ability to freshen breath naturally, peppermint is a favorite with people everywhere. Peppermint essential oil is often listed as one of the most useful essential oils available, and its ability to address a wide range of ailments makes it a valuable addition to your natural medicine collection.

APPLICATION METHODS

- Use in the bath or shower for absorption and aromatherapy benefits
- Diffuse for aromatherapy benefits
- Massage, diluted, for physical ailments
- Neat for headache and severe muscle pain and stiffness
- Use with compress for muscle pain and stiffness

BLENDS WITH

- Basil
- Benzoin
- Black pepper
- Cinnamon
- Cypress
- Dill
- Eucalyptus
- Geranium
- Grapefruit
- Juniper
- Lavender
- Lemon
- Lemon eucalyptus
- Manuka
- Marjoram
- Niaouli
- Pine
- Rose geranium
- Rosemary
- Spearmint
- Tea tree

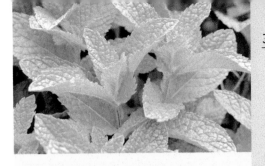

PRECAUTIONS

Peppermint essential oil can be a dermal irritant for sensitive individuals. Conduct a patch test before use. Peppermint essential oil irritates the mucus membranes. This essential oil helps in some cases of indigestion, but it can make acid reflux, GERD, and heartburn worse in many instances. Those with epilepsy should avoid peppermint essential oil. Because it can stimulate menstrual flow, pregnant women should avoid peppermint essential oil.

- Avoid contact with mucus membranes.
- Do not use if you are pregnant.
- Do not use if you have epilepsy.
- May cause skin irritation.
- Not safe for children under 6.

REPEL INSECTS NATURALLY WITH PEPPERMINT.
Several studies published by the U.S. National Library of Medicine show that peppermint is effective in repelling insects, including flies. One study in the *Medical and Veterinary Entomology* journal showed that dairy cattle, which normally attract high numbers of flies, experienced a 75 percent reduction in fly activity when treated with a solution made of sunflower oil and peppermint essential oil.

MEDICINAL USES

Analgesic

Antibacterial

Anti-
inflammatory

Antifungal

Antimicrobial

Antiseptic

Asthma

Depression

Expectorant

Fatigue

Fever

Flatulence

Headache

Indigestion

Insecticide

Insect repellant

Intestinal
parasites

Mental
alertness

Muscle pain
and stiffness

Nausea

Ringworm

Scabies

Sedative

Sinus infection

Sunburn

Vertigo

Petitgrain *Citrus aurantium*

Sometimes referred to as bitter orange, petitgrain essential oil has a gorgeous aroma that many people find irresistible. Often used to formulate natural remedies for depression, it is also useful in combating insomnia, acne, and many other common ailments.

APPLICATION METHODS

- Use in the bath or shower for absorption and aromatherapy benefits
- Diffuse for aromatherapy benefits
- Massage, diluted, for physical ailments
- Use with compress for muscle pain and stiffness

BLENDS WITH

- Aniseed
- Benzoin
- Bergamot
- Cardamom
- Cedarwood
- Cinnamon
- Clary sage
- Clove
- Coriander
- Cypress
- Eucalyptus
- Frankincense
- Geranium
- Jasmine
- Juniper
- Lavender
- Lemon
- Mandarin
- Manuka
- Marjoram
- Melissa
- Neroli
- Nutmeg
- Orange
- Oregano
- Palmarosa
- Patchouli
- Rose
- Rosemary
- Rosewood
- Sandalwood
- Tangerine
- Valerian
- Ylang-ylang

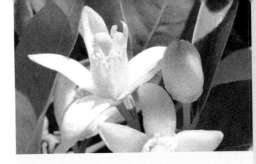

PRECAUTIONS

Petitgrain essential oil has a deeply relaxing effect and should not be used prior to driving, operating machinery, or doing other tasks that require concentration.

- May act as a sedative.

MEDICINAL USES

Acne

Addiction

Anger

Antibacterial

Antiseptic

Anxiety

Depression

Insomnia

Muscle relaxant

Nervousness

Oily skin

Relaxation

Stomach flu

Stress

Pine   *Pinus sylvestris*

Just as the scent of fresh evergreen branches is invigorating yet relaxing, pine essential oil energizes the mind while easing pain and relaxing the body. One of the best essential oils for easing muscle pain, arthritis, and rheumatism, pine is also ideal for use when combating a cold or the flu.

APPLICATION METHODS

- Use in the bath or shower for absorption and aromatherapy benefits
- Diffuse for aromatherapy benefits
- Massage, diluted, for physical ailments
- Use with compress for muscle pain and stiffness

BLENDS WITH

- Bay
- Bergamot
- Cedarwood
- Citronella
- Clary sage
- Cypress
- Eucalyptus
- Fennel
- Fir needle
- Frankincense
- Grapefruit
- Juniper
- Lavandin
- Lavender
- Lemon eucalyptus
- Manuka
- Marjoram
- Myrrh
- Oregano
- Peppermint
- Rosemary
- Sandalwood
- Spikenard
- Spruce
- Tea tree
- Thyme
- Valerian

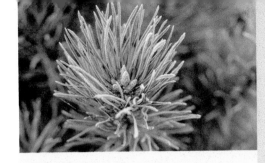

PRECAUTIONS

Pine essential oil can be a dermal irritant for sensitive individuals. Conduct a patch test before use.

- Do not use if you are pregnant.
- May cause skin irritation.
- Not safe for children under 6.

MEDICINAL USES

Analgesic	Fatigue
Antibacterial	Flu
Antifungal	Hangover
Anti-inflammatory	Infection
	Insecticide
Antimicrobial	Insect repellant
Antiseptic	Intestinal
Antiviral	parasites
Arthritis	Joint pain
Asthma	Laryngitis
Bactericidal	Mental
Bronchitis	alertness
Cellulite	Muscle pain
Circulatory	and stiffness
health	Nervousness
Cold	Prostatitis
Cough	Rheumatism
Decongestant	Sinus infection
Disinfectant	Stress
Diuretic	Tendinitis
Expectorant	Tennis elbow

Rose   *Rosa x damascena*

The scent of roses is wonderfully relaxing, and rose essential oil is even more so. Useful for treating problem skin and other ailments, its greatest value lies in its emotional benefits. Whether you are grieving, suffering from depression, or dealing with a toddler who is prone to temper tantrums, rose essential oil can help.

APPLICATION METHODS

- Use in the bath or shower for absorption and aromatherapy benefits
- Diffuse for aromatherapy benefits
- Massage, diluted, for physical ailments
- Neat for problem skin
- Use with compress for muscle pain and stiffness

BLENDS WITH

- Bay
- Benzoin
- Bergamot
- Cedarwood
- Cinnamon
- Clary sage
- Clove
- Fennel
- Frankincense
- Geranium
- German chamomile
- Ginger
- Jasmine
- Lavender
- Lemon
- Mandarin
- Melissa
- Myrrh
- Orange
- Palmarosa
- Patchouli
- Petitgrain
- Roman chamomile
- Rose geranium
- Rosewood
- Sandalwood
- Spikenard
- Tangerine
- Vetiver
- Ylang-ylang

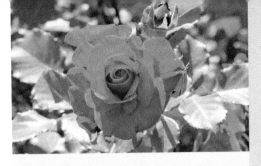

PRECAUTIONS

Due to the cost and desirability of rose essential oil, it is often adulterated. Ensure you purchase it from a trusted source. Because it can stimulate menstrual flow, pregnant women should avoid rose essential oil.

- Do not use if you are pregnant.

EXPERIENCE THE FRAGRANCE OF 60 ROSES IN A SINGLE DROP OF ESSENTIAL OIL. An average of 60 roses goes into every single drop of rose essential oil, and just one ounce contains about 60,000 roses. A very small amount of this essential oil goes a long way, so use it judiciously to defray cost.

MEDICINAL USES

Anger
Antiallergenic
Anti-inflammatory
Antiseptic
Antiviral
Anxiety
Aphrodisiac
Asthma
Bactericidal
Broken or swollen capillaries
Calming
Circulatory health
Depression

Dermatitis
Eczema
Grief
Headache
Menstrual support
Nervousness
PMS
PTSD
Relaxation
Rosacea
Sprains and strains
Stress
Temper tantrums

Rose Geranium   *Pelargonium graveolens*

There are approximately 700 geranium species, but only one of them produces this delightfully scented essential oil. A wonderful alternative to geranium essential oil, it has a crisp rather than overly sweet floral aroma. It is useful for a wide range of ailments, and it will prove to be a valuable addition to your essential oil collection.

APPLICATION METHODS

- Use in the bath or shower for absorption and aromatherapy benefits
- Diffuse for aromatherapy benefits
- Massage, diluted, for physical ailments
- Use with compress for muscle pain and stiffness

BLENDS WITH

- Allspice
- Basil
- Bay
- Bergamot
- Cajeput
- Carrot seed
- Cedarwood
- Citronella
- Clary sage
- Clove
- Cypress
- Fennel
- Geranium
- German chamomile
- Ginger
- Grapefruit
- Jasmine
- Juniper
- Lavender
- Lemon
- Lemon eucalyptus
- Lime
- Mandarin
- Myrrh
- Neroli
- Orange
- Palmarosa
- Patchouli
- Peppermint
- Roman chamomile
- Rose
- Rosemary
- Rosewood
- Sandalwood
- Ylang-ylang

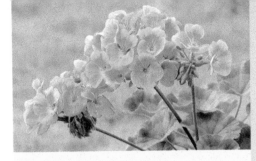

PRECAUTIONS

- Do not use if you are pregnant.

MEDICINAL USES

Aging skin

Antiseptic

Anxiety

Balances hormones

Bruise

Burn

Cellulite

Depression

Detoxification

Diuretic

Eczema

Edema

Hemorrhoids

Insect repellent

Intestinal parasites

Lice

Menstrual support

PMS

Ringworm

Shingles

Skin care

Stress

Wounds

Wrinkles

Rosemary   *Rosmarinus officinalis*

Rosemary is one of the world's most popular medicinal plants, and for good reason. It is useful in numerous applications, ranging from stimulating hair growth to staving off infection. Rosemary essential oil has a crisp fragrance that appeals to nearly everyone, and its uses are almost limitless.

APPLICATION METHODS

- Use in the bath or shower for absorption and aromatherapy benefits
- Diffuse for aromatherapy benefits
- Massage, diluted, for physical ailments
- Use with compress for muscle pain and stiffness

BLENDS WITH

- Basil
- Bay
- Bergamot
- Birch
- Black pepper
- Calamus
- Camphor
- Cassia
- Cedarwood
- Cinnamon
- Citronella
- Clary sage
- Elemi
- Eucalyptus
- Fennel
- Fir needle
- Frankincense
- Geranium
- German chamomile
- Grapefruit
- Helichrysum
- Hyssop
- Juniper
- Lavandin
- Lavender
- Lemon
- Lemon eucalyptus
- Lemongrass
- Lime
- Manuka
- Marjoram
- Myrrh
- Niaouli
- Nutmeg
- Oregano
- Peppermint
- Petitgrain
- Pine
- Rose geranium
- Sage
- Spearmint
- Spruce
- Tea tree
- Thyme
- Valerian

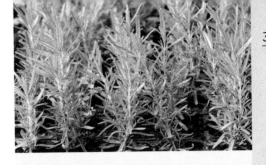

PRECAUTIONS

Those with epilepsy or hypertension should avoid rosemary essential oil. Because it can stimulate menstrual flow, pregnant women should avoid rosemary essential oil.

- Do not use if you are pregnant.
- Do not use if you have epilepsy.
- Do not use if you have hypertension.

MEDICINAL USES

Aging skin
Analgesic
Antibacterial
Antiseptic
Aphrodisiac
Arthritis
Asthma
Bronchitis
Cellulite
Cold
Cough
Circulatory
   health
Decongestant
Depression
Disinfectant
Diuretic
Expectorant
Flu

Fungicide
Gout
Hair growth
Intestinal
   parasites
Joint pain
Laryngitis
Memory
Menstrual
   support
Mental
   alertness
Migraine
Muscle pain
   and stiffness
Rheumatism
Sinus infection
Varicose veins

Rosewood *Aniba rosaeodora*

Consider trying rosewood essential oil if you have aging or injured skin, or if you tend to suffer from depression or seasonal affective disorder. This fragrant essential oil is more costly than most and does not treat a large number of ailments; however, it does an impressive job in favorably affecting a select few.

APPLICATION METHODS

- Use in the bath or shower for absorption and aromatherapy benefits
- Diffuse for aromatherapy benefits
- Massage, diluted, for physical ailments
- Use with a compress for muscle pain and stiffness

BLENDS WITH

- Aniseed
- Bergamot
- Geranium
- Jasmine
- Lemon
- Lime
- Orange
- Petitgrain
- Rose
- Rose geranium
- Sage
- Sandalwood
- Ylang-ylang

PRECAUTIONS

Rosewood essential oil is generally considered safe.

HEAL YOUR WOUNDS AND RELAX WITH ROSEWOOD ESSENTIAL OIL. Rosewood essential oil has such a distinctive aroma that the pursuit of this product by the perfume and soap manufacturers caused deforestation in the 1990s. A study published in *Ethnopharmacology* in 2009 found that this oil has a relaxing sedative effect on people when inhaled. Beyond the signature scent, rosewood oil can regenerate tissues, making it an effective wound, blemish, and wrinkle treatment when applied undiluted.

MEDICINAL USES

Aging skin

Analgesic

Antiseptic

Aphrodisiac

Bactericidal

Cold

Cough

Depression

Emotional balance

Fever

Flu

Headache

Impotence

Insecticide

Low testosterone

Nausea

Seasonal affective disorder

Wrinkles

Sage *Salvia officinalis*

Perhaps best known for adding savory flavor to food, sage has a long history of use in herbal medicine. Sage essential oil proves particularly useful for solving skin problems, addressing menstrual issues and PMS, and helping alleviate menopausal symptoms. Its medicinal properties make it a valuable addition to your natural apothecary.

APPLICATION METHODS

- Use in the bath or shower for absorption and aromatherapy benefits
- Diffuse for aromatherapy benefits
- Massage, diluted, for physical ailments
- Use with compress for muscle pain and stiffness

BLENDS WITH

- Black pepper
- Elemi
- Hyssop
- Lavandin
- Lavender
- Lemon
- Lemon eucalyptus
- Manuka
- Rosemary
- Rosewood

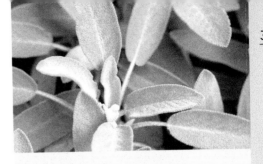

PRECAUTIONS

Do not use sage essential oil internally. Those with epilepsy should avoid sage essential oil. Sage essential oil can be a dermal irritant for sensitive individuals. Conduct a patch test before use. Because it can stimulate menstrual flow, pregnant women should avoid sage essential oil.

- Do not use if you are pregnant.
- Do not use if you have epilepsy.
- May cause skin irritation.
- Not safe for internal use.

COMBAT FUNGUS WITH SAGE. Sage essential oil is widely used in traditional medicine. A 2013 study reported by the medical journal *BioMed Research International* showed that sage essential oil demonstrates antifungal activity against dermatophytes, and did not damage skin cells.

MEDICINAL USES

Antibacterial	Memory
Antifungal	Menopause
Anti-inflammatory	support
	Menstrual
Antimicrobial	support
Antioxidant	Mental
Antiseptic	alertness
Depression	Muscle pain
Dermatitis	and stiffness
Disinfectant	PMS
Diuretic	Psoriasis
Fever	Rheumatism
Grief	Ringworm
Insecticide	Scabies
Insect repellant	Skin care
Jock itch	Wounds
Laxative	

Sandalwood *Santalum album*

People have been using sandalwood for more than 4,000 years. Always prized for its marvelous, exotic fragrance, sandalwood essential oil is an excellent choice for problem skin as well as for treating a wide range of ailments, from chest colds to urinary tract infections.

APPLICATION METHODS

- Use in the bath or shower for absorption and aromatherapy benefits
- Diffuse for aromatherapy benefits
- Gargle for sore throat
- Massage, diluted, for physical ailments
- Use with compress for muscle pain and stiffness

BLENDS WITH

- Benzoin
- Bergamot
- Birch
- Black pepper
- Cardamom
- Cedarwood
- Citronella
- Clary sage
- Clove
- Coriander
- Fennel
- Frankincense
- Geranium
- Ginger
- Jasmine
- Lavender
- Lemon
- Mandarin
- Manuka
- Myrrh
- Neroli
- Orange
- Palmarosa
- Patchouli
- Petitgrain
- Pine
- Rose
- Rose geranium
- Rosewood
- Tangerine
- Vetiver
- Ylang-ylang

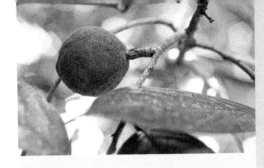

PRECAUTIONS

Sandalwood essential oil has a deeply relaxing effect and should not be used prior to driving, operating machinery, or doing other tasks that require concentration.

- May act as a sedative.

MEDICINAL USES

Aging skin

Anger

Anti-inflammatory

Antiseptic

Aphrodisiac

Asthma

Bronchitis

Calming

Chest infection

Cold

Cough

Depression

Eczema

Irritability

Meditation

Nervousness

Scarring

Sedative

Skin care

Sore throat

Urinary tract infection

Wounds

Wrinkles

Spearmint *Mentha spicata*

Milder than peppermint, spearmint essential oil has a sweet, minty fragrance that makes it ideal for use in applications that range from formulating household cleaners to diffusing for naturally fresh indoor air. Safe for children, it may be used to replace peppermint essential oil in many instances.

APPLICATION METHODS

- Use in the bath or shower for absorption and aromatherapy benefits
- Diffuse for aromatherapy benefits
- Massage, diluted, for physical ailments
- Use with compress for muscle pain and stiffness

BLENDS WITH

- Basil
- Benzoin
- Dill
- Eucalyptus
- Jasmine
- Lavender
- Lemon
- Orange
- Peppermint
- Rosemary

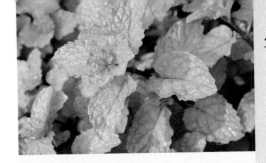

PRECAUTIONS

- Avoid use with homeopathic remedies.

MEDICINAL USES

Acne	Dental health
Analgesic	Diuretic
Anesthetic	Expectorant
Antibacterial	Fever
Anti-inflammatory	Flatulence
	Headache
Antiseptic	Hiccups
Antispasmodic	Indoor air freshener
Asthma	
Bronchitis	Laryngitis
Clarity	Migraine
Cold	Muscle pain and stiffness
Colic	
Cough	Nausea
Decongestant	Sinus infection

Spikenard   *Nardostachys jatamansi*

Many people have heard of or used valerian, but few have tried spikenard, which is a close relative to the stronger herb. Often referred to as Indian valerian, spikenard is of particular use for treating insomnia and nervousness; this essential oil is also of great value in skin care solutions and natural perfumes.

APPLICATION METHODS

- Use in the bath or shower for absorption and aromatherapy benefits
- Diffuse for aromatherapy benefits
- Massage, diluted, for physical ailments
- Use with compress for muscle pain and stiffness

BLENDS WITH

- Clary sage
- Clove
- Cypress
- Frankincense
- Geranium
- Juniper
- Lavender
- Lemon
- Myrrh
- Neroli
- Palmarosa
- Patchouli
- Pine
- Rose
- Vetiver

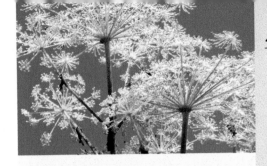

PRECAUTIONS

Spikenard essential oil has a deeply relaxing effect and should not be used prior to driving, operating machinery, or doing other tasks that require concentration.

- May act as a sedative.

MEDICINAL USES

Aging skin

Antiallergenic

Antibiotic

Antifungal

Anti-inflammatory

Antiseptic

Bactericidal

Circulatory health

Colic

Constipation

Fungicidal

Insomnia

Laxative

Menstrual support

Migraine

Nausea

Nervousness

PMS

Rash

Sedative

Skin care

Stress

Tension

Varicose veins

Spruce   *Tsuga canadensis*

Spruce essential oil has a sweet evergreen fragrance that most people find irresistible. Not only is it a marvelous oil for diffusing to freshen indoor air naturally, it proves particularly useful for treating arthritis, infections, and muscle pain, among other common ailments.

APPLICATION METHODS

- Use in the bath or shower for absorption and aromatherapy benefits
- Diffuse for aromatherapy benefits
- Massage, diluted, for physical ailments
- Use with compress for muscle pain and stiffness

BLENDS WITH

- Benzoin
- Cedarwood
- Clary sage
- Lavender
- Pine
- Rosemary

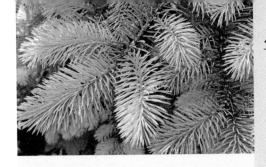

PRECAUTIONS

Spruce essential oil can be a dermal irritant for sensitive individuals. Conduct a patch test before use.

- May cause skin irritation.

MEDICINAL USES

Antimicrobial

Antiseptic

Arthritis

Bronchitis

Cold

Cough

Diuretic

Expectorant

Flu

Indoor air freshener

Infection

Laryngitis

Meditation

Muscle pain and stiffness

Relaxation

Rheumatism

Stress

Tagetes   *Tagetes minuta*

If you are looking for a potent insect repellent that doubles as an addition to your natural medicine arsenal, consider tagetes essential oil. This sweet-smelling oil is sourced from an herb that is closely related to the marigold, and it may also be used to speed the healing of minor wounds.

APPLICATION METHODS

- Use in the bath or shower for absorption and aromatherapy benefits
- Diffuse for aromatherapy benefits
- Massage, diluted, for physical ailments
- Use with compress for muscle pain and stiffness

BLENDS WITH

- Bergamot
- Clary sage
- Jasmine
- Lavender
- Lemon
- Orange

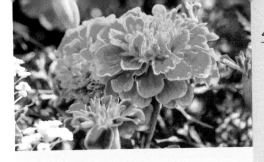

PRECAUTIONS

Tagetes essential oil can be a dermal irritant for sensitive individuals. Conduct a patch test before use. Blend with care, as this is a very powerful essential oil. Tagetes essential oil is phototoxic. Avoid exposing application sites to sunlight for 12 to 24 hours following application. Because it can stimulate menstrual flow, pregnant women should avoid tagetes essential oil.

- Avoid exposure to sunlight for 12 to 24 hours after use.
- Do not use if you are pregnant.
- May cause skin irritation.

MEDICINAL USES

Antibiotic

Antifungal

Antimicrobial

Bactericidal

Bronchitis

Bunion

Callus

Chest infection

Cold

Cough

Insecticide

Insect repellent

Wounds

Tangerine   *Citrus reticulata*

The tangerine is a cultivar of the mandarin orange, and as such, the essential oils have similar properties. Their fragrances are somewhat different; try both to see which appeals to you more.

APPLICATION METHODS

- Use in the bath or shower for absorption and aromatherapy benefits
- Diffuse for aromatherapy benefits
- Massage, diluted, for physical ailments
- Use with compress for muscle pain and stiffness

BLENDS WITH

- Basil
- Black pepper
- Cinnamon
- Clary sage
- Clove
- Fennel
- Frankincense
- Geranium
- German chamomile
- Grapefruit
- Jasmine
- Juniper
- Lemon
- Myrrh
- Neroli
- Nutmeg
- Palmarosa
- Patchouli
- Petitgrain
- Roman chamomile
- Rose
- Sandalwood
- Ylang-ylang

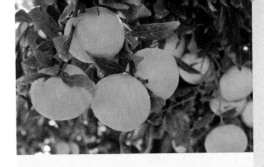

PRECAUTIONS

Tangerine essential oil can be a dermal irritant for sensitive individuals. Conduct a patch test before use. Tangerine essential oil is phototoxic. Avoid exposing application sites to sunlight for 12 to 24 hours following application.

- Avoid exposure to sunlight for 12 to 24 hours after use.
- May cause skin irritation.

MEDICINAL USES

Acne	Mood booster
Antimicrobial	Nervousness
Antiseptic	Oily hair
Cold	Oily skin
Constipation	Scars
Cough	Sedative
Diarrhea	Skin care
Disinfectant	Stimulant
Diuretic	Stress
Flatulence	Stretch marks
Flu	Temper tantrums
Hypnotic	Tension
Insomnia	Wrinkles
Laxative	

Tea Tree *Melaleuca alternifolia*

Tea tree is one of the most useful essential oils available, as it treats a wide range of ailments with swift efficiency. Also referred to as melaleuca, this essential oil is useful in formulating household cleansers, cleaning wounds, and eliminating fungal infections.

APPLICATION METHODS

- Use in the bath or shower for absorption and aromatherapy benefits
- Diffuse for aromatherapy benefits
- Massage, diluted, for physical ailments
- Neat for fungal infections and wounds
- Use with compress for muscle pain and stiffness

BLENDS WITH

- Basil
- Bergamot
- Black pepper
- Calamus
- Clary sage
- Clove
- Cypress
- Eucalyptus
- Geranium
- German chamomile
- Helichrysum
- Juniper
- Lavender
- Lemon
- Lemon eucalyptus
- Lemongrass
- Manuka
- Marjoram
- Myrrh
- Niaouli
- Nutmeg
- Oregano
- Peppermint
- Pine
- Ravensara
- Roman chamomile
- Rosemary
- Thyme
- Ylang-ylang

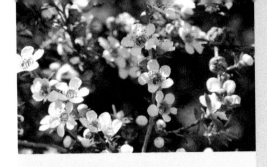

PRECAUTIONS

Do not use tea tree essential oil internally. It can be a dermal irritant for sensitive individuals. Conduct a patch test before use.

- May cause skin irritation.
- Not safe for internal use.

MEDICINAL USES

Abscess	Disinfectant
Acne	Expectorant
Analgesic	Flu
Animal bite	Fungicidal
Antibacterial	Jock itch
Antifungal	Immune
Anti-inflammatory	stimulant
	Insecticide
Antimicrobial	Insect repellent
Antiseptic	Intestinal
Antiviral	parasites
Arthritis	Laryngitis
Athlete's foot	Oily hair
Bedsores	Oily skin
Boil	Rash
Bronchitis	Ringworm
Burn	Sinus infection
Cold	Skin tags
Cough	Sunburn
Cradle cap	Thrush
Dandruff	Wart
Decongestant	Whooping
Dental health	cough
Diaper rash	Wounds

Thyme   *Thymus vulgaris*

Thyme is one of the oldest medicinal plants on record, and continues to offer a number of benefits to those who prefer to use natural remedies. In addition to its usefulness as an antiseptic, it helps ease pain, comfort those suffering from sports injuries, and speed up natural childbirth.

APPLICATION METHODS

- Use in the bath or shower for absorption and aromatherapy benefits
- Diffuse for aromatherapy benefits
- Gargle for dental health, sore throat, and tonsillitis
- Massage, diluted, for physical ailments
- Neat to animal bites and wounds
- Use with compress for muscle pain and stiffness

BLENDS WITH

- Bay
- Bergamot
- Cajeput
- Cinnamon
- Eucalyptus
- Grapefruit
- Helichrysum
- Lavandin
- Lavender
- Lemon
- Lemon eucalyptus
- Lemongrass
- Manuka
- Marjoram
- Oregano
- Pine
- Rosemary
- Tea tree

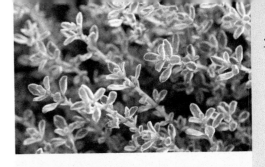

PRECAUTIONS

Thyme essential oil can be a dermal irritant for sensitive individuals. Conduct a patch test before use. Thyme essential oil irritates the mucus membranes. Because it can stimulate menstrual flow, pregnant women should avoid thyme essential oil.

- Avoid contact with mucus membranes.
- Do not use if you are pregnant.
- May cause skin irritation.

MEDICINAL USES

Animal bite	Flu
Antiseptic	Gout
Bactericidal	Insecticide
Boil	Intestinal
Bronchitis	parasites
Bruise	Memory
Childbirth	Muscle pain
Cold	and stiffness
Cough	Rheumatism
Dental health	Sore throat
Depression	Sprains and
Dermatitis	strains
Diuretic	Tonsillitis
Eczema	Weight-loss
Edema	support
Expectorant	

Valerian *Valeriana officinalis*

If you suffer from restlessness or are looking for an effective natural sleep aid, valerian essential oil is a must-have. It is also useful for alleviating stress, and can be beneficial to those suffering from restless legs syndrome.

APPLICATION METHODS

- Use in the bath or shower for absorption and aromatherapy benefits
- Diffuse for aromatherapy benefits
- Massage, diluted, for physical ailments
- Use with compress for muscle pain and stiffness

BLENDS WITH

- Cedarwood
- Lavender
- Mandarin
- Patchouli
- Petitgrain
- Pine
- Rosemary

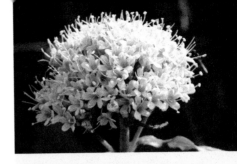

PRECAUTIONS

Valerian essential oil can be a dermal irritant for sensitive individuals. Conduct a patch test before use. Valerian essential oil has a deeply relaxing effect and should not be used prior to driving, operating machinery, or doing other tasks that require concentration. Because it can stimulate menstrual flow, pregnant women should avoid valerian essential oil.

- Do not use if you are pregnant.
- May act as a sedative.
- May cause skin irritation.
- Not safe for children under 6.

MEDICINAL USES

Anxiety

Bactericidal

Depression

Diuretic

Emotional balance

Fever

Headache

Insomnia

Menstrual support

Nervousness

Restless legs syndrome

Restlessness

Sedative

Stress

Teeth grinding

Tendinitis

Vetiver   *Vetiveria zizanoides*

Vetiver is a balancing essential oil for body and mind alike. Sourced from the roots of a tropical grass, it has an earthy, somewhat herbaceous fragrance that is likely to remind you of the scent of a forest during autumn. Use it to alleviate emotional upset, calm anger, treat dry and aging skin, and ease aches and pains.

APPLICATION METHODS

- Use in the bath or shower for absorption and aromatherapy benefits
- Diffuse for aromatherapy benefits
- Massage, diluted, for physical ailments
- Neat for painful areas and problem skin
- Use with compress for muscle pain and stiffness

BLENDS WITH

- Bergamot
- Black pepper
- Cardamom
- Cedarwood
- Clary Sage
- Coriander
- Frankincense
- Geranium
- Ginger
- Grapefruit
- Helichrysum
- Jasmine
- Lavender
- Lemon
- Lemon eucalyptus
- Lemongrass
- Mandarin
- Myrrh
- Orange
- Patchouli
- Rose
- Sandalwood
- Spikenard
- Ylang-ylang

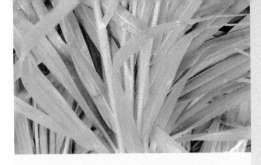

PRECAUTIONS

Vetiver essential oil has a deeply relaxing effect and should not be used prior to driving, operating machinery, or doing other tasks that require concentration.

- May act as a sedative.

INCREASE FOCUS WITH VETIVER. A 2012 study reported by the journal *Biomedical Research* showed that participants who inhaled vetiver essential oil while focusing on visually demanding tasks were able to react faster than those who were not exposed to vetiver. Use this essential oil to stay on track while studying and working on mentally challenging tasks.

MEDICINAL USES

Absent-mindedness	Insomnia
Acne	Intestinal parasites
ADD/ADHD	Joint stiffness
Aging skin	Meditation
Analgesic	Menstrual support
Anger	Muscle pain and stiffness
Antibacterial	
Antifungal	Muscular dystrophy
Anti-inflammatory	
Antimicrobial	Oily hair
Antiseptic	Oily skin
Anxiety	Pancreatitis
Arthritis	Postpartum depression
Autism	
Circulatory health	Sedative
	Skin care
Cramping	Stress
Depression	Tendinitis
Emotional balance	Tennis elbow
	Wounds
Hyperactivity	Wrinkles

Ylang-Ylang   *Cananga odorata*

With an enticing, intoxicating fragrance that promotes mental and emotional balance, ylang-ylang essential oil is one of the best for easing anger, depression, and stress. It is also an excellent essential oil for balancing skin and hair, and its hypotensive quality makes it ideal for use by those suffering from high blood pressure and associated ailments.

APPLICATION METHODS

- Use in the bath or shower for absorption and aromatherapy benefits
- Diffuse for aromatherapy benefits
- Massage, diluted, for physical ailments
- Use with compress for muscle pain and stiffness

BLENDS WITH

- Allspice
- Bay
- Bergamot
- Black pepper
- Calamus
- Cardamom
- Cinnamon
- Clary sage
- Clove
- Coriander
- Cypress
- Fennel
- Frankincense
- Geranium
- German chamomile
- Ginger
- Grapefruit
- Helichrysum
- Jasmine
- Lemon
- Lemon eucalyptus
- Lemongrass
- Lime
- Mandarin
- Myrrh
- Neroli
- Orange
- Palmarosa
- Patchouli
- Petitgrain
- Roman chamomile
- Rose
- Rose geranium
- Rosewood
- Sandalwood
- Tangerine
- Tea tree
- Vetiver

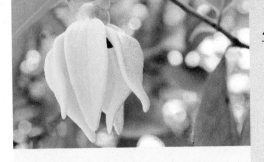

PRECAUTIONS

Excessive use of ylang-ylang essential oil may cause nausea and headaches in sensitive individuals. Use moderately for best results. Ylang-ylang essential oil has a deeply relaxing effect and should not be used prior to driving, operating machinery, or doing other tasks that require concentration.

- May act as a sedative.
- May cause headaches.

CALM DOWN NATURALLY WITH YLANG-YLANG.
Ylang-ylang essential oil has been proven to significantly increase calmness when inhaled. In a study reported in the January 2008 *International Journal of Neuroscience*, test subjects exposed to ylang-ylang essential oil experienced decreased alertness and increased relaxation, while those exposed to peppermint essential oil became more alert.

MEDICINAL USES

Anger	Flu
Antibacterial	Grief
Antifungal	Hair growth
Anti-inflammatory	Heart health
Antiseptic	Hypertension
Anxiety	Impotence
Aphrodisiac	Insomnia
Cold	Itchiness
Cough	Low testosterone
Dandruff	Meditation
Depression	Nervousness
Diabetes	Oily hair
Disinfectant	Oily skin
Dry hair	Sedative
Expectorant	Skin care
Fatigue	Stress

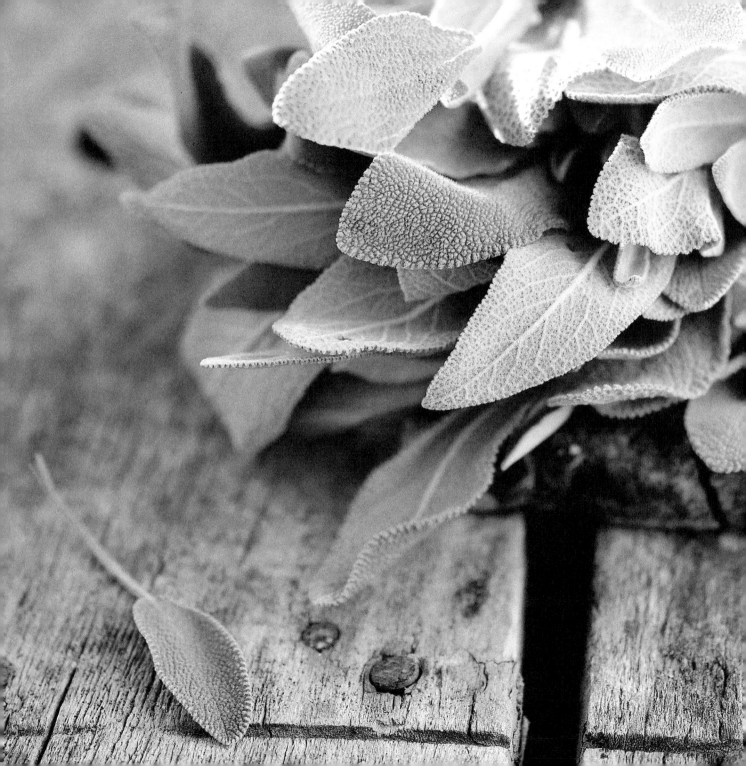

GLOSSARY

abortifacient: Any substance capable of inducing an abortion. This includes any substance that may cause miscarriage at any stage of pregnancy.

adulterate: A term used to describe the mixing of pure essential oils with another substance. An essential oil is deemed to be adulterated when it has been watered down but sold as 100 percent essential oil.

allergy: A general term for an irritation caused by contact with an irritant or allergen. Allergens can be introduced via inhalation, skin contact, or ingestion.

analgesic: A substance that relieves or deadens pain. Many analgesic drugs are narcotics; analgesic essential oils are non-narcotic.

anthelmintic: A substance capable of expelling or destroying intestinal parasites. This type of substance is also referred to as a vermifuge.

antibacterial: A substance that slows the growth of bacteria. In some cases, this term refers to a substance that prevents bacteria.

antidepressant: A substance that helps counteract the symptoms of mild depression. Many essential oils possess this quality.

antifungal: A substance that slows or prevents the growth of fungi. Many antifungal essential oils are as effective as commercial antifungal agents.

antihistamine: A substance that counteracts the body's natural reactions to allergens. Most commercial antihistamines cause undesirable side effects.

antimicrobial: A substance that reduces microbial activity. Antimicrobial essential oils are particularly useful for household cleansers.

antiseptic: A substance that helps slow or stop infection. Applying an antiseptic shortly after an injury helps speed healing.

antispasmodic: A substance that helps stop muscle spasms and cramping. Antispasmodic essential oils are useful in treating digestive issues, menstrual cramps, and muscle pain caused by cramping.

aphrodisiac: A substance that increases sexual desire. In some cases, aphrodisiacs may help improve sexual function.

aromatherapy: The practice of using natural aromatic substances, including essential oils, for their physical and psychological therapeutic benefits.

astringent: A substance that causes organic tissue to contract.

bactericidal: A substance that kills or destroys bacteria. Most bactericidal essential oils are ideal for external use and for formulating nontoxic household cleansers.

botanical name: A specific Latin name that distinguishes variants of plants that share the same common name.

carrier oil: An oil used for diluting an essential oil prior to use. Examples include apricot kernel, grape seed, olive, and sweet almond oils.

common name: A plant's "everyday" name. For example, there are several different species of plants that fall under the common name *orange*.

detoxifier: A substance that aids in detoxifying the body. Detoxifiers work by facilitating the removal of impurities from organs, tissue, or the bloodstream.

dilution: The act of making an essential oil less potent by adding a carrier oil.

diffuser: A device used for releasing essential oil molecules into the air. Various models are available commercially. Be sure to follow the manufacturer's directions.

diuretic: A substance that removes water from the body while stimulating urine production. When using diuretics of any kind, it is vital that you drink plenty of water.

expectorant: A substance that aids in the expulsion of mucus from the lungs. In most cases, expectorants prompt productive coughing.

febrifuge: A substance that helps reduce fevers. Using a cold compress with a febrifuge can help hasten fever reduction.

food grade: An essential oil considered safe for use in food by the FDA.

fragrance: An aroma. Products labeled as fragrances are derived by synthetic means and are not essential oils.

fungicide: A substance that destroys fungi. Fungicidal essential oils are useful for topical application as well as for formulating nontoxic household cleansers.

germicide: A substance that destroys germs. Germicidal essential oils are useful for formulating remedies as well as for diffusing; when diffused, they promote clean, healthy indoor air.

hemostatic: A substance that helps stop bleeding. Most hemostatic substances work by helping blood clot faster.

herbal: Pertaining to plants.

hypertension: High blood pressure. The term is typically used when discussing long-term high blood pressure rather than acute high blood pressure.

insoluble: A substance that is not capable of being dissolved in liquid such as water.

laxative: A substance that promotes bowel movements. Most commercial laxatives are unnecessarily harsh.

narcotic: A substance that promotes sleep. Most narcotics produce deep, heavy sleep.

neat: Undiluted. Some essential oils are suitable for using neat, while others are not. As you delve deeper into the world of essential oils, you will notice that some practitioners are much more conservative than others, advising readers not to use undiluted essential oils. The choice is yours.

pathogen: A substance that causes or produces a disease. Most pathogens are viruses or bacteria.

pendant: A necklace made from a variety of materials, such as glass or terra-cotta, that you can add your favorite essential oil to and wear throughout the day.

rectification: The process of re-distilling certain essential oils to rid them of undesirable constituents.

single oil: An essential oil from only one plant species. Examples are clary sage, clove, geranium, and sweet orange. Some literature refers to these oils as *single notes*.

soluble: A substance that is capable of being dissolved in liquid such as water.

styptic: A substance that helps stop external bleeding. Styptics are most useful for treating small wounds.

synthetic: A substance that is unnatural or created in a laboratory. Many commercially produced drugs are synthetic.

volatile: A substance that is unstable and evaporates easily.

AILMENTS & OILS QUICK REFERENCE GUIDE

AILMENT	SUGGESTED ESSENTIAL OILS	METHODS OF APPLICATION
Aches and pains	basil, benzoin, black pepper, chamomile (German or Roman), cinnamon, clove, cypress, ginger, juniper, lavender, marjoram, rosemary, thyme, ylang-ylang	bath, compress, massage
Acne	basil, bergamot, cedarwood, cypress, geranium, grapefruit, lavender, palmarosa, rose, rose geranium, tea tree	bath, massage, neat
Aging skin	frankincense, geranium, rose, rose geranium, sandalwood	bath, compress, massage, neat
Anxiety	basil, bergamot, cedarwood, clary sage, frankincense, jasmine, lavender, orange, patchouli, rose	bath, inhalation, massage, vaporization
Arthritis	basil, eucalyptus, frankincense, peppermint, pine, rosemary	bath, compress, massage
Asthma	chamomile (German or Roman), eucalyptus, frankincense, myrrh, pine	bath, inhalation, massage, vaporization
Athlete's foot	clove, lavender, lemon, myrrh, tea tree	bath, massage, neat
Bug bites	basil, cinnamon, lemon, lavender, tea tree	neat
Burn	carrot seed, lavender, tea tree	bath, neat
Chest congestion	benzoin, camphor, eucalyptus, frankincense, myrrh, peppermint, niaouli, pine, rosemary, tea tree, thyme	bath, inhalation, massage, vaporization
Chilblains	benzoin, black pepper, cedarwood, ginger, juniper, thyme	bath, compress, massage
Colds and flu	basil, benzoin, black pepper, camphor, cinnamon, eucalyptus, ginger, lavender, lemon, niaouli, peppermint, pine, tea tree, thyme	bath, inhalation, massage, vaporization
Constipation	black pepper, clary sage, cypress, eucalyptus, peppermint, rosemary	bath, compress, massage
Cramps	chamomile (German or Roman), lavender, sandalwood, vetiver	bath, compress, massage
Dandruff	cedarwood, lavender, lemongrass, sandalwood, tea tree	hair products

AILMENT	SUGGESTED ESSENTIAL OILS	METHODS OF APPLICATION
Dental health	clove, frankincense, myrrh, peppermint	gargle, neat, oil pulling
Diarrhea	chamomile (German or Roman), lavender, rose, neroli	bath, compress, massage
Ear infections / swimmer's ear	basil, frankincense, myrrh, tea tree	neat
Eczema	benzoin, chamomile (German or Roman), frankincense, lavender, myrrh, sandalwood, vetiver	bath, massage
Fluid retention	black pepper, cypress, grapefruit, juniper, lemon, lime, orange	bath, compress, massage
Hay fever	bergamot, cedarwood, chamomile (German or Roman), eucalyptus, geranium, lavender, lemongrass, pine, rose, rose geranium, rosemary, rosewood, ylang-ylang	bath, inhalation, massage, vaporization
Headache	chamomile (German or Roman), lavender, lemongrass, peppermint, rosewood	bath, inhalation, massage, vaporization
Head lice	bergamot, eucalyptus, geranium, lavender, lemon, rose geranium, tea tree	hair products
Indigestion	dill, fennel, ginger, lemon, mandarin, peppermint	inhalation, massage
Insomnia	chamomile (German or Roman), lavender, orange, ylang-ylang	bath, inhalation, massage
Nausea	bergamot, black pepper, chamomile (German or Roman), fennel, ginger, grapefruit, lavender, mandarin, orange, peppermint, rosewood	bath, inhalation, vaporization
Sprains	chamomile (German or Roman), eucalyptus, geranium, lavender, pine	bath, compress, massage
Throat infection / sore throat	basil, benzoin, black pepper, cinnamon, eucalyptus, lavender, lemon, niaouli, peppermint, pine, sandalwood, tea tree	bath, compress, gargle, inhalation, massage, vaporization
Weight loss / metabolism	grapefruit, lemon, patchouli	inhalation
Wounds	chamomile (German or Roman), frankincense, geranium, helichrysum, hyssop, lavender, patchouli, rose geranium, tea tree	bath, compress, neat

RESOURCES

Abu-Darwish, M. S., C. Cabral, I. V. Ferreira, M. J. Gonçalves, C. Cavaleiro, M. T. Cruz, T. H. Al-bdour, and L. Salgueiro. "Essential Oil of Common Sage (*Salvia officinalis L.*) from Jordan: Assessment of Safety in Mammalian Cells and Its Antifungal and Anti-inflammatory Potential." *BioMed Research International* (October 2013). doi:10.1155/2013/538940.

Adukwu, E. C., S. C. H. Allen, and C. A. Phillips. "The Anti-biofilm Activity of Lemongrass (*Cymbopogon flexuosus*) and Grapefruit (*Citrus paradisi*) Essential Oils against Five Strains of *Staphylococcus aureus*." *Journal of Applied Microbiology* 113, no. 5 (November 2012): 1217–27. doi:10.1111/j.1365-2672.2012.05418.x.

Aura Cacia. Accessed May 23, 2014. http://www.auracacia.com/.

Białoń, M., T. Krzyśko-Łupicka, M. Koszałkowska, and P. P. Wieczorek. "The Influence of Chemical Composition of Commercial Lemon Essential Oils on the Growth of *Candida* Strains." *Mycopathologia* 177 (2014): 29–39. doi:10.1007/s11046-013-9723-3.

Callan, Nancy W., Mal P. Westcott, Susan Wall-MacLane, James B. Miller, Leon Welty, and Louise Strang. "German Chamomile." Montana State University. Accessed May 23, 2014. http://ag.montana.edu/warc/research/horticulture/chamomile.htm.

Caprigem8387. "Aromatherapy Positively Affects Mood, EEG Patterns of Alertness." StudyMode.com. May 2007. http://www.studymode.com/essays/Aromatherapy-Positively-Affects-Mood-Eeg-Patterns-115154.html.

Cooksley, Virginia Gennari. *Aromatherapy: A Lifetime Guide to Healing with Essential Oils*. Englewood Cliffs, New Jersey: Prentice Hall, 1996.

Dias, M. I., J. C. Barreira, R. C. Calhelha, M. J. Queiroz, M. B. Oliveira, M. Soković, and I. C. Ferreira. "Two-Dimensional PCA Highlights the Differentiated Antitumor and Antimicrobial Activity of Methanolic and Aqueous Extracts of *Laurus nobilis L.* from Different Origins." *BioMed Research International* (April 2014). doi:10.1155/2014/520464.

dōTerra. Accessed May 23, 2014. http://www.doterra.com/.

Edwards, Victoria H. *The Aromatherapy Companion: Medicinal Uses/Ayurvedic Healing/Body-Care Blends/Perfumes & Scents/Emotional Health & Well-Being.* North Adams, MA: Storey Publishing, 1999.

Eksteins, Angela. "Beware: Adulteration of Essential Oils, Part I." *Natural News.* December 5, 2009. http://www.naturalnews.com/027661_essential_oils_adulteration.html#.

Essential Oil Joy. "Cassia." Accessed July 25, 2014. http://essentialoiljoy.com/cassia/.

Falsetto, Sharon. "Scientific Testing of Essential Oils." Decoded Science. December 19, 2012. http://www.decodedscience.com/scientific-testing-of-essential-oils/22544.

Fink, Sheri. "The Deadly Choices at Memorial." *New York Times.* August 25, 2009. http://www.nytimes.com/2009/08/30/magazine/30doctors.html?pagewanted=all&_r=0.

Gladstar, Rosemary. *Rosemary Gladstar's Medicinal Herbs: A Beginner's Guide.* North Adams, MA: Storey Publishing, 2012.

Heritage Essential Oils. Accessed May 23, 2014. http://heritageessentialoils.com/.

Hotta, Mariko, Rieko Nakata, Michiko Katsukawa, Kazuyuki Hori, Saori Takahashi, and Hiroyasu Inoue. "Carvacrol, a Component of Thyme Oil, Activates PPARalpha and gamma and Suppresses COX-2 Expression." *Journal of Lipid Research* 51 (January 2010): 132–9. doi:10.1194/jlr.M900255-JLR200.

Inshanti. "*Eucalyptus globulus.*" Accessed July 25, 2014. http://www.inshanti.com/essential-oils-products/451/eucalyptus-globulus-eucalyptus-globulus-2.

International Fragrance Association. Accessed May 23, 2014. http://www.ifraorg.org/.

Jafarzadeh, Mehdi, Soroor Arman, and Fatemeh Farahbakhsh Pour. "Effect of Aromatherapy with Orange Essential Oil on Salivary Cortisol and Pulse Rate in Children during Dental Treatment: A Randomized Controlled Clinical Trial." *Advanced Biomedical Research* 2 (March 2013). doi:10.4103/2277-9175.107968.

Johnson, Scott A. *Surviving When Modern Medicine Fails: A Definitive Guide to Essential Oils That Could Save Your Life During a Crisis.* Amazon Digital Services, Inc., 2013. Kindle edition.

Ju, M. S., S. Lee, I. Bae, M. H. Hur, K. Seong, and M. S. Lee. "Effects of Aroma Massage on Home Blood Pressure, Ambulatory Blood Pressure, and Sleep Quality in Middle-Aged Women with Hypertension." *Evidence-Based Complementary and Alternative Medicine* (January 2013). doi:10.1155/2013/403251.

Keville, Kathi, and Mindy Green. *Aromatherapy: A Complete Guide to the Healing Art.* New York: Crossing Press, 2009.

Kim, I. H., C. Kim, K. Seong, M. H. Hur, H. M. Lim, and M. S. Lee. "Essential Oil Inhalation on Blood Pressure and Salivary Cortisol Levels in Prehypertensive and Hypertensive Subjects." *Evidence-Based Complementary and Alternative Medicine* (November 2012). doi:10.1155/2012/984203.

Lachance, S., and G. Grange. "Repellent Effectiveness of Seven Plant Essential Oils, Sunflower Oil and Natural Insecticides against Horn Flies on Pastured Dairy Cows and Heifers." *Medical and Veterinary Entomology* 28, no. 2 (June 2014): 193–200. doi:10.1111/mve.12044.

Langreth, Robert. "Drug Prices Soar for Top-Selling Brands." *Bloomberg*. May 1, 2014. http://www.bloomberg.com/infographics/2014-05-01/drug-prices-soar-for-top-selling-brands.html.

Lawless, Julia. *The Illustrated Encyclopedia of Essential Oils*. Rockport, MA: Element, 1995.

Lis-Balchin, Maria. *Aromatherapy Science: A Guide for Healthcare Professionals*. Grayslake, IL: Pharmaceutical Press, 2006.

Locke, Tim. "Smelling Rosemary 'May Improve Memory.'" WebMD. April 9, 2013. http://www.webmd.boots.com/news/20130409/smelling-rosemary-may-improve-memory.

Lodhia, M. H., K. R. Bhatt, and V. S. Thaker. "Antibacterial Activity of Essential Oils from Palmarosa, Evening Primrose, Lavender, and Tuberose." *Indian Journal of Pharmaceutical Sciences* 71, no. 2 (March 2009): 134–6. doi:10.4103/0250-474X.54278.

Matsubara, E., K. Shimizu, M. Fukagawa, Y. Ishizi, C. Kakoi, T. Hatayama, J. Nagano, T. Okamoto, K. Ohnuki, and R. Kondo. "Volatiles Emitted from the Roots of *Vetiveria zizanioides* Suppress the Decline in Attention during a Visual Display Terminal Task." *Biomedical Research* 33, no. 5 (2012): 299–308. http://www.ncbi.nlm.nih.gov/pubmed/23124250.

Matthys, H., C. de Mey, C. Carls, A. Ryś, A. Geib, and T. Wittig. "Efficacy and Tolerability of Myrtol Standardized in Acute Bronchitis: A Multi-Centre, Randomised, Double-Blind, Placebo-Controlled Parallel Group Clinical Trial vs. Cefuroxime and Ambroxol." *Arzneimittelforschung* 50, no. 8 (August 2000): 700–11. http://www.ncbi.nlm.nih.gov/pubmed/10994153.

Mayo Clinic. "Heartburn Causes." May 21, 2011. http://www.mayoclinic.org/diseases-conditions/heartburn-gerd/basics/causes/CON-20019545.

McNeill, K. P., P. Byers, T. Kittle, S. Hand, J. Parham, L. Mena, C. Blackmore, et al. "Surveillance for Illness and Injury after Hurricane Katrina—Three Counties, Mississippi, September 5 to October 11, 2005." *Morbid and Mortality Weekly Report (MMWR)*. Centers for Disease Control and Prevention. Accessed May 21, 2014. http://www.cdc.gov/mmwr/preview/mmwrhtml/mm5509a2.htm.

Merck Manual for Health Care Professionals. "Drug Absorption." Last modified May 2014. http://www.merckmanuals.com/professional/clinical_pharmacology/pharmacokinetics/drug_absorption.html.

Moss, M., S. Hewitt, L. Moss, and K. Wesnes. "Modulation of Cognitive Performance and Mood by Aromas of Peppermint and Ylang-Ylang." *International Journal of Neuroscience* 118, no. 1 (January 2008): 59–77. http://www.ncbi.nlm.nih.gov/pubmed/18041606/.

Mountain Rose Herbs. Accessed May 23, 2014. https://www.mountainroseherbs.com/.

Native American Nutritionals. Accessed May 23, 2014. http://www.nativeamericannutritionals.com/.

National Cancer Institute at the National Institutes of Health. "Aromatherapy and Essential Oils." Last modified October 16, 2012. http://www.cancer.gov/cancertopics/pdq/cam/aromatherapy/patient.

Now Foods. Accessed May 23, 2014. http://www.nowfoods.com/.

Oboh, G., A. O. Ademosun, O. V. Odubanjo, and I. A. Akinbola. "Antioxidative Properties and Inhibition of Key Enzymes Relevant to Type 2 Diabetes and Hypertension by Essential Oils from Black Pepper." *Advances in Pharmacological Sciences* (November 2013). doi:10.1155/2013/926047.

Ohno, T., M. Kita, Y. Yamaoka, S. Imamura, T. Yamamoto, S. Mitsufuji, T. Kodama, K. Kashima, and J. Imanishi. "Antimicrobial Activity of Essential Oils against *Helicobacter pylori.*" *Helicobacter* 8, no. 3 (June 2003): 207–15. http://www.ncbi.nlm.nih.gov/pubmed/12752733. Accessed June 13, 2014.

Opalchenova, G., and D. Obreshkova. "Comparative Studies on the Activity of Basil—an Essential Oil from Ocimum basilicum L.—against Multidrug Resistant Clinical Isolates of the Genera Staphylococcus, Enterococcus and Pseudomonas by Using Different Test Methods." *Journal of Microbiological Methods* 54, no. 1 (July 2003): 105–10. http://www.ncbi.nlm.nih.gov/pubmed?Db=pubmed&Cmd=ShowDetailView&TermToSearch=12732427.

Parker-Pope, Tara. "Rare Infection Prompts Neti Pot Warning." *The Well Column. New York Times.* September 3, 2012. http://well.blogs.nytimes.com/2012/09/03/rare-infection-prompts-neti-pot-warning/.

Pasay, C., K. Mounsey, G. Stevenson, R. Davis, L. Arlian, M. Morgan, D. Vyszenski-Moher, K. Andrews, and J. McCarthy. "Acaricidal Activity of Eugenol Based Compounds against Scabies Mites." *PLoS One* 5, no. 8 (August 2010). doi:10.1371/journal.pone.0012079.

Power, Joie. "Inhaling Essential Oils: Essential Oils and the Sense of Smell." Aromatherapy School. Accessed May 26, 2014. http://www.aromatherapy-school.com/aromatherapy-schools/aromatherapy-articles/inhaling-essential-oils.html.

Ravensthorpe, Michael. "Studies Show That Oil Pulling Can Kill Harmful Bacteria in the Mouth." *Natural News*. May 29, 2014. http://www.naturalnews.com/045343_oil_pulling_harmful_bacteria_oral_health.html.

Rocky Mountain Oils. Accessed May 23, 2014. http://www.rockymountainoils.com/.

Rokbeni, N., Y. M'rabet, S. Dziri, H. Chaabane, M. Jemli, X. Fernandez, and A. Boulila. "Variation of the Chemical Composition and Antimicrobial Activity of the Essential Oils of Natural Populations of Tunisian Daucus carota L. (Apiaceae)." *Chemistry and Biodiversity* 10, no. 12 (December 2013): 2278–90. doi:10.1002/cbdv.201300137.

Sagon, Candy. "AARP Study Finds Popular Brand-Name Drug Prices Far Outstrip Inflation." American Association of Retired Persons. August 25, 2010. http://www.aarp.org/health/drugs-supplements/info-08-2010/aarp_study_finds_prices_of_popular_brandname_drugs_far_outstrip_inflation.html.

Salmalian, H., R. Saghebi, A. A. Moghadamnia, A. Bijani, M. Faramarzi, F. Nasiri Amiri, F. Bakouei, F. Behmanesh, and R. Bekhradi. "Comparative Effect of *Thymus vulgaris* and Ibuprofen on Primary Dysmenorrhea: A Triple-Blind Clinical Study." *Caspian Journal of Internal Medicine* 5, no. 2 (2014): 82–8. http://www.ncbi.nlm.nih.gov/pubmed/24778782.

Sartorelli, P., A. D. Marquioreto, A. Amaral-Baroli, M. E. Lima, and P. R. Moreno. "Chemical Composition and Antimicrobial Activity of the Essential Oils from Two Species of Eucalyptus." *Phytotherapy Research* 21, no. 3 (March 2007): 231–3. http://www.ncbi.nlm.nih.gov/pubmed/17154233.

Stansbury, Jillian. "Photosensitizing Herbs." *Naturopathic Doctor News and Review* (NDNR). May 1, 2011. http://ndnr.com/naturopathic-news/photosensitizing-coumarins-for-skin-diseases-and-cancers/.

Starwest Botanicals. Accessed May 23, 2014. http://www.starwest-botanicals.com/.

Stiles, K. G., "Shelf Life of Essential Oils." Health Mastery Systems. Accessed May 23, 2014. http://www.kgstiles.com/article-shelf-life-4/.

Thompson, A., D. Meah, N. Ahmed, R. Conniff-Jenkins, E. Chileshi, C. O. Phillips, T. C. Claypole, D. W. Forman, and P. E. Row. "Comparison of the Antibacterial Activity of Essential Oils and Extracts of Medicinal and Culinary Herbs to Investigate Potential New Treatments for Irritable Bowel Syndrome." *BMC Complementary and Alternative Medicine* (November 2013). doi:10.1186/1472-6882-13-338.

Tisserand, Robert. "Aromatherapy." Accessed July 25, 2014. http://roberttisserand.com/about/aromatherapy/

———. "Lemon on the Rocks: Keep Your Essential Oils Cool." *I'm Just Saying . . .* (blog). July 26, 2013. http://roberttisserand.com/2013/07/lemon-on-the-rockskeep-your-essential-oils-cool/.

Tumen, I., I. Süntar, F. J. Eller, H. Keleş, and E. K. Akkol. "Topical Wound-Healing Effects and Phytochemical Composition of Heartwood Essential Oils *of Juniperus virginiana L., Juniperus occidentalis* Hook, and *Juniperus ashei* J. Buchholz." *Journal of Medicinal Food* 16, no. 1 (January 2013): 48–55. doi:10.1089/jmf.2012.2472.

University of Maryland Medical Center. "Aloe." Last modified May 7, 2013. http://umm.edu/health/medical/altmed/herb/aloe.

———. "Bronchitis." Last modified May 7, 2013. http://umm.edu/health/medical/altmed/condition/bronchitis.

———. "Ginger." Last modified July 31, 2013. http://umm.edu/health/medical/altmed/herb/ginger.

———. "Tension Headache." Last modified May 7, 2013. http://umm.edu/health/medical/altmed/condition/tension-headache.

USDA (United States Department of Agriculture). "Organic Agriculture." Last modified April 11, 2014. http://www.usda.gov/wps/portal/usda/usdahome?contentid=organic-agriculture.html.

Waple, Anne. "Hurricane Katrina." National Oceanic and Atmospheric Administration's National Climatic Data Center. December 2005. http://www1.ncdc.noaa.gov/pub/data/extremeevents/specialreports/Hurricane-Katrina.pdf.

WebMD. "Genital Herpes Health Center." Accessed June 5, 2014. http://www.webmd.com/genital-herpes/pain-management-herpes.

White, Gregory Lee. *Essential Oils and Aromatherapy: How to Use Essential Oils for Beauty, Health, and Spirituality*. White Willow Books, 2013. Kindle edition.

Wildwood, Chrissie. *The Encyclopedia of Aromatherapy*. Rochester, VT: Healing Arts Press, 1996.

Wong, Cathy. "Health Benefits of Black Walnut." About.com. Last modified July 7, 2014. http://altmedicine.about.com/od/herbsupplementguide/a/Black-Walnut.htm.

Worwood, Valerie Ann. *The Complete Book of Essential Oils and Aromatherapy: Over 600 Natural, Non-Toxic, and Fragrant Recipes to Create Health—Beauty—A Safe Home Environment*. Novato, CA: New World Library, 1991.

———. *The Fragrant Mind: Aromatherapy for Personality, Mind, Mood, and Emotion*. Novato, CA: New World Library, 1996.

Young Living. Accessed May 23, 2014. http://www.youngliving.com/en_US.

KNOW YOUR ESSENTIAL OIL BRANDS

There are many excellent essential oil brands available, but it can be difficult to determine which are widely trusted. To make that task easier, here are ten of the most popular.

AURA CACIA

Description: Founded in 1982, Aura Cacia offers an extensive line of essential oils and products containing essential oils.

Where to Buy: You can purchase Aura Cacia products online and in select stores. Many retail locations carry only a portion of the essential oils the company produces.

Ratings and Reviews: Customers give Aura Cacia high marks for its reasonable prices and for the quality of the essential oils they produce.

DŌTERRA

Description: dōTerra was founded in 2008, making it a relatively new company. dōTerra offers numerous single oils as well as several signature blends and kits containing an array of the most popular oils and blends.

Where to Buy: You can purchase dōTerra essential oils only from independent product consultants, either in person or online. Many dōTerra consultants sell on Amazon, eBay, and similar sites.

Ratings and Reviews: dōTerra receives high marks for quality but lower marks for pricing. The company's kits receive excellent reviews.

Other: Use caution when purchasing dōTerra essential oils online. Some consumers have reported that they've received fake products from certain sellers, so check seller ratings before placing an order.

EDENS GARDEN

Description: Edens Garden offers a good selection of essential oil singles, synergistic blends, and carrier oils. Starter kits are also available.

Where to Buy: You can purchase Edens Garden essential oils online.

Ratings and Reviews: Customers give this company high marks for quality, price, and service.

Other: Use caution if purchasing Edens Garden products from anywhere other than their website or another official storefront, such as Amazon. Products labeled as Edens Garden that are purchased from another seller may be adulterated or overpriced.

HERITAGE ESSENTIAL OILS

Description: Heritage Essential Oils is a small family-owned company that provides a good selection of single essential oils, blends, and products made with essential oils. Custom blends are available, as are organic essential oils and wild-crafted essential oils.

Where to Buy: You can purchase Heritage Essential Oils online.

Ratings and Reviews: Customers give this company high marks for quality and value.

MOUNTAIN ROSE HERBS

Description: Mountain Rose Herbs has been offering certified organic products since 1987. An extensive selection of single essential oils are available along with blended oils and products containing them.

Where to Buy: You can purchase Mountain Rose Essential Oils at the company's website and at its headquarters, located in Eugene, Oregon. You may find a selection of these essential oils at a local retailer, as well.

Ratings and Reviews: Customers give Mountain Rose Herbs excellent marks for quality, price, and ease of ordering.

Other: This company offers a loyalty program and student discounts.

NATIVE AMERICAN NUTRITIONALS

Description: Native American Nutritionals offers an extensive array of single essential oils, blends, and products containing essential oils. This small company focuses on providing organic products.

Where to Buy: You can purchase Native American Nutritionals essential oils online and from the company's catalog, which can be ordered online. Some health food stores carry the products, as well.

Ratings and Reviews: Customers give Native American Nutritionals high marks for prices, quality, and selection.

Other: Native American Nutritionals offers a 30-day guarantee on their products.

NOW FOODS

Description: NOW Foods has been producing natural foods and other supplements since 1948. The company offers a vast array of products, including numerous essential oils, carrier oils, and products containing essential oils.

Where to Buy: You can purchase NOW Foods essential oils at some major retailers and online.

Ratings and Reviews: Customers give NOW Foods essential oils good marks for price and quality. These oils are often eclipsed by those offered by smaller companies when compared side by side.

ROCKY MOUNTAIN OILS

Description: Rocky Mountain Oils offers an extensive array of essential oils, blends, and products containing essential oils. Kits and samplers are also available.

Where to Buy: You can purchase Rocky Mountain Oils essential oils online and in some retail locations. The company also offers a printed catalog.

Ratings and Reviews: Rocky Mountain Oils has earned excellent marks from customers, particularly as they offer small sampler kits that allow first-time users to try a selection of oils without making a large investment.

Other: Rocky Mountain Oils has a customer satisfaction guarantee.

STARWEST BOTANICALS

Description: Starwest Botanicals offers a wide selection of the most popular essential oils as well as several organic essential oils and essential oil blends. The company has been in business since 1975; today, they are among the largest suppliers of organic herbs and essential oils in the United States.

Where to Buy: You can purchase Starwest Botanicals essential oils online and in some health food stores.

Ratings and Reviews: Customers give Starwest Botanicals rave reviews for quality and price.

Other: Starwest Botanicals offers a 100 percent money-back guarantee in the event a customer is unhappy with an essential oil for any reason.

YOUNG LIVING

Description: Young Living offers several single essential oils, a wide selection of popular blends, and products that contain essential oils.

Where to Buy: You can purchase Young Living essential oils online and from independent distributors.

Ratings and Reviews: Some people take exception to the fact that Young Living is a multi-level marketing company; however, the products themselves receive high marks for quality. Customers are particularly satisfied with the company's blended oils.

AILMENTS INDEX

OILS INDEX

INDEX

CPSIA information can be obtained
at www.ICGtesting.com
Printed in the USA
LVOW06s1155121016
508303LV00001B/1/P